TOP TRAILS™

Lake Tahoe

50 MUST-DO HIKES FOR EVERYONE

Written by

Mike White

 **WILDERNESS PRESS** ... *on the trail since 1967*

Top Trails Lake Tahoe: 50 Must-Do Hikes for Everyone
3rd Edition

Copyright © 2015 by Mike White

All photos, except where noted, © by Mike White
Maps: Mike White and Scott McGrew
Cover design: Frances Baca Design and Scott McGrew
Text design: Frances Baca Design

Library of Congress Cataloging-in-Publication Data

White, Michael C., 1952-
Top trails Lake Tahoe : must-do hikes for everyone / written by Mike White. — 3rd edition.
   pages cm
   ISBN 978-0-89997-777-5 (paperback) — ISBN 0-89997-777-4 (pbk.)
   1. Hiking—Tahoe, Lake, Region (Calif. and Nev.)—Guidebooks. 2. Trails—Tahoe, Lake,
Region (Calif. and Nev.)—Guidebooks. 3. Tahoe, Lake, Region (Calif. and Nev.)—Guidebooks. I. Title. II. Title: Lake Tahoe.
   GV199.42.T16W55 2015
   796.5109794›38—dc23

                              2015008840

ISBN 978-0-89997-777-5; eISBN: 978-0-89997-778-2

Manufactured in the United States of America

Published by: **Wilderness Press**
               An imprint of Keen Communications, LLC
               2204 First Avenue South, Suite 102
               Birmingham, AL 35233
               800-443-7227
               info@wildernesspress.com
               wildernesspress.com

Visit our website for a complete listing of our books and for ordering information.

Distributed by Publishers Group West

Cover photo: Eagle Falls (see Trail 26) © Celso Diniz

SAFETY NOTICE: Although Keen Communications/Wilderness Press and the author
have made every attempt to ensure that the information in this book is accurate at press
time, they are not responsible for any loss, damage, injury, or inconvenience that may occur to anyone while using this book. You are responsible for your own safety and health
while in the wilderness. The fact that a trail is described in this book does not mean that
it will be safe for you. Be aware that trail conditions can change from day to day. Always
check local conditions, know your own limitations, and consult a map and compass.

The Top Trails™ Series

Wilderness Press

When Wilderness Press published *Sierra North* in 1967, no other trail guide like it existed for the Sierra backcountry. The first print run sold out in less than two months, and its success heralded the beginning of Wilderness Press. Since we were founded almost 50 years ago, we have expanded our territories to cover California, Alaska, Hawaii, the US Southwest, the Pacific Northwest, the Midwest, the Southeast, New England, Canada, and Baja California.

Wilderness Press continues to publish comprehensive, accurate, and readable outdoor books. Hikers, backpackers, kayakers, skiers, snowshoers, climbers, cyclists, and trail runners rely on Wilderness Press for accurate outdoor adventure information.

Top Trails

In its Top Trails guides, Wilderness Press has paid special attention to organization so that you can find the perfect hike each and every time. Whether you're looking for a steep trail to test yourself on or a walk in the park, a romantic waterfall or a city view, Top Trails will lead you there.

Each Top Trails guide contains trails for everyone. The trails selected provide a sampling of the best that the region has to offer. These are the must-do hikes, walks, runs, and bike rides, with every feature of the area represented.

Every book in the Top Trails series offers:

- The Wilderness Press commitment to accuracy and reliability
- Ratings and rankings for each trail
- Distances and approximate times
- Easy-to-follow trail notes
- Map and permit information

TRAIL FEATURES TABLE

Lake Tahoe Trails

TRAIL NUMBER AND NAME	Page	Difficulty -12345+	Length in Miles	Type	Hiking	Running	Mountain Biking	Horses	Child-Friendly	Dogs Allowed	Wheelchair Access	Permit
1. North Tahoe												
1 Mount Lola and White Rock Lake	28	4	14.4	↗	✓	✓	✓	✓		✓		
2 Sagehen Creek	33	1	5.0	↗	✓	✓	✓	✓	✓	✓		
3 Summit Lake, Frog Lake Overlook, and Warren Lake	37	1–5	4.0–15.0	↗	✓			✓		✓		
4 Castle Peak	43	5	9.6	↗	✓					✓		
5 Castle Valley, Round Valley, and Andesite Peak	48	3	9.6	↺	✓	✓	✓	✓	✓	✓		
6 Loch Leven Lakes	54	4	8.0	↗	✓	✓	✓	✓		✓		
7 Mount Judah Loop	60	3	4.6	↺	✓	✓		✓	✓	✓		
8 PCT: Donner Pass to Squaw Valley	65	5	15.0	↘	✓			✓				
9 Granite Chief	72	5	10.2	↗	✓							
10 Five Lakes Basin	78	3	4.0	↗	✓	✓				✓		
11 TRT: Tahoe City to Truckee River Canyon Viewpoint	82	4	11.4	↗	✓	✓	✓	✓		✓		
12 Mount Rose	86	3	10.0	↗	✓	✓				✓		
13 Rim to Reno Trail	92	5	18.0	↘	✓	✓				✓		
14 Tahoe Meadows Nature Trails	99	1	0.8–3.3	↺	✓	✓			✓	✓	✓	
15 TRT: Tahoe Meadows to Brockway Summit	105	5	19.5	↘	✓	✓	✓			✓		
16 TRT: Tahoe Meadows to Twin Lakes	115	4	19.0	↗	✓	✓	✓	✓		✓		
2. West Tahoe												
17 TRT: Ward Creek to Twin Peaks	130	3	11.6	↗	✓	✓	✓	✓		✓		
18 PCT: Barker Pass to Twin Peaks	135	4	11.2	↗	✓	✓	✓			✓		
19 Ellis Lake and Ellis Peak	139	4	8.6	↗	✓	✓	✓			✓		
20 Bear Pen	144	4	13.4	↗	✓	✓		✓	✓			
21 General Creek Trail to Lost and Duck Lakes	148	3	13.0	↗	✓	✓	✓	✓	✓			
22 Ed Z'berg Sugar Pine Point State Park Nature Trails	153	1	0.25–1.7	↺	✓				✓		✓	

TRAIL FEATURES TABLE

	TERRAIN				Lake or Shore		FLORA & FAUNA			EXPOSURE			OTHER				
Canyon	Mountain	Summit	Stream	Waterfall	Lake or Shore	Autumn Colors	Wildflowers	Birds	Wildlife	Cool & Shady	Great Views	Photo Opportunity	Camping	Secluded	Historical Interest	Geologic Interest	Steep
✓	✓	✓	✓		✓		✓				✓	✓	✓	✓			
✓			✓			✓	✓	✓	✓			✓					
✓	✓				✓			✓			✓	✓	✓				✓
✓	✓	✓					✓				✓	✓					
✓	✓	✓					✓		✓		✓		✓		✓		✓
✓	✓				✓		✓					✓	✓				
	✓	✓									✓						
	✓	✓									✓	✓	✓	✓			
✓	✓	✓	✓		✓			✓		✓	✓	✓					
✓	✓				✓							✓					
											✓	✓					✓
	✓	✓	✓	✓			✓				✓	✓					
✓	✓		✓	✓		✓	✓				✓	✓	✓				
	✓		✓				✓	✓	✓		✓	✓					
	✓	✓		✓	✓		✓	✓			✓	✓	✓	✓			
	✓						✓	✓			✓	✓	✓				
✓	✓	✓	✓	✓			✓				✓	✓					
	✓	✓			✓		✓	✓			✓	✓					
	✓	✓			✓						✓	✓	✓				✓
✓			✓				✓						✓	✓			
✓	✓		✓		✓					✓	✓		✓	✓			
					✓		✓		✓	✓	✓						

TRAIL FEATURES TABLE

Lake Tahoe Trails

USES & ACCESS

Trail Number and Name	Page	Difficulty 1-2345+	Length in Miles	Type	Hiking	Running	Mountain Biking	Horses	Child-Friendly	Dogs Allowed	Wheelchair Access	Permit
3. South Tahoe												
23 TYT: Meeks Bay to Tallant Lakes	170	4	16.0	↗	✓	✓		✓		✓		
24 D. L. Bliss State Park: Rubicon Point and Lighthouse Loop	175	1	2.0	○	✓				✓			
25 Rubicon Trail	179	2	5.0	↘	✓				✓			
26 Vikingsholm and Eagle Falls	184	2	2.5	↗	✓				✓		✓	
27 Eagle Lake	189	2	2.0	↗	✓	✓			✓	✓		✓
28 Bayview Trail to Velma Lakes	194	4	10.5	○	✓	✓		✓		✓		✓
29 Cascade Falls	199	1	1.5	↗	✓	✓		✓	✓	✓		✓
30 Taylor Creek Visitor Center Nature Trails	203	1	up to 1.1	↗	✓				✓		✓	
31 Mount Tallac	208	5	9.4	↗	✓	✓				✓		✓
32 Glen Alpine to Susie and Heather Lakes and Lake Aloha	213	4	11.8	↗	✓	✓		✓		✓		✓
33 Triangle Lake, Echo Peak, and Angora Lakes Loop	218	5	7.2	○	✓							✓
34 Echo Lakes to Lake Aloha	225	2–3	7.6–12.6	↗	✓	✓		✓	✓	✓		✓
35 Echo Lake to Lake of the Woods and Ropi Lake	230	3–4	8.0–13.0	↗	✓	✓	✓		✓	✓		✓
36 Ralston Peak	235	4	6.0	↗	✓	✓				✓		✓
37 Horsetail Falls	239	3	3.0	↗	✓							✓
38 Big Meadow to Carson Pass	244	3	10.4	↘	✓	✓		✓		✓		
39 Upper Blue Lake to Fourth of July Lake	250	4	9.0	↗	✓			✓		✓		✓
40 Winnemucca and Round Top Lakes Loop	255	3	4.8	○	✓	✓		✓		✓		✓
41 Emigrant Lake	261	3	8.2	↗	✓	✓		✓		✓		✓
42 Thunder Mountain	265	3	8.5	↗	✓	✓	✓	✓		✓		
4. East Tahoe												
43 TRT: Spooner Summit to Snow Valley Peak	278	4	12.4	↗	✓	✓		✓		✓		
44 Spooner Lake	283	1	1.8	○	✓	✓			✓	✓	✓	
45 Marlette Lake	287	3	9.0	↗	✓	✓		✓		✓		
46 Flume Trail	292	3	13.0	↘			✓					
47 TRT: Spooner Summit to South Camp Peak	297	3	10.2	↗	✓	✓	✓	✓		✓		
48 Skunk Harbor	302	3	3.2	↗	✓	✓	✓		✓			
49 TRT: Kingsbury South to Star Lake	306	4	17.6	↗	✓	✓	✓			✓		
50 TRT: Armstrong Pass to Star Lake	311	3	12.8	↗	✓	✓	✓	✓		✓		

| | TERRAIN | | | | FLORA & FAUNA | | | | | EXPOSURE | | | OTHER | | | | |
Canyon	Mountain	Summit	Stream	Waterfall	Lake or Shore	Autumn Colors	Wildflowers	Birds	Wildlife	Cool & Shady	Great Views	Photo Opportunity	Camping	Secluded	Historical Interest	Geologic Interest	Steep
✓	✓		✓		✓		✓					✓	✓				
					✓						✓	✓					
					✓						✓	✓					
				✓	✓				✓	✓	✓	✓			✓		
✓	✓		✓	✓	✓							✓	✓			✓	
✓	✓		✓		✓		✓					✓	✓				
			✓	✓									✓				
			✓		✓		✓	✓	✓		✓	✓			✓		
✓	✓	✓	✓		✓		✓				✓	✓					
✓	✓		✓	✓	✓		✓				✓	✓	✓				
✓	✓	✓			✓		✓			✓	✓	✓					✓
	✓				✓		✓					✓	✓				
✓	✓	✓	✓	✓	✓	✓	✓	✓	✓	✓			✓				
✓	✓	✓					✓				✓	✓		✓			✓
✓	✓		✓	✓							✓	✓				✓	
✓	✓		✓		✓	✓	✓	✓	✓			✓	✓	✓	✓		
✓					✓		✓	✓	✓		✓	✓	✓				
✓	✓		✓		✓		✓					✓	✓		✓		
✓	✓		✓		✓		✓			✓		✓	✓				
	✓	✓						✓			✓	✓					
	✓	✓				✓		✓		✓	✓	✓					
	✓				✓	✓	✓	✓	✓			✓			✓		
✓	✓		✓		✓	✓	✓	✓	✓			✓					
✓	✓				✓	✓					✓	✓					
	✓	✓					✓				✓	✓					
					✓		✓				✓	✓			✓		
	✓				✓						✓	✓	✓	✓			
	✓	✓			✓						✓	✓	✓				

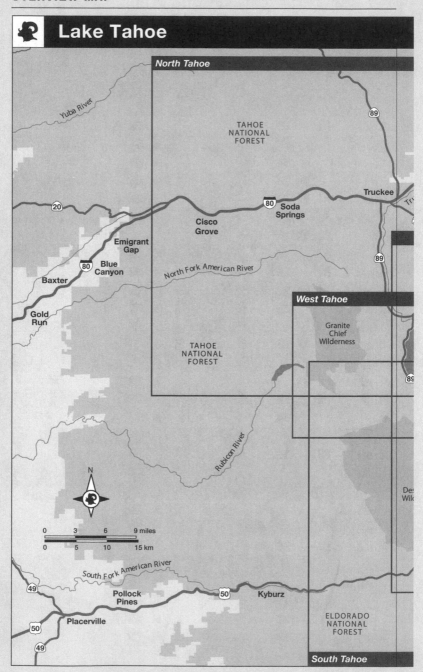

Lake Tahoe

North Tahoe

Yuba River

TAHOE
NATIONAL
FOREST

89

Truckee

20

80 Soda
Springs

Cisco
Grove

Emigrant
Gap

89

80 Blue
Canyon

Baxter

North Fork American River

West Tahoe

Gold
Run

Granite
Chief
Wilderness

TAHOE
NATIONAL
FOREST

89

Rubicon River

N

0   3   6   9 miles
0   5   10   15 km

Des
Wild

South Fork American River

49

Pollock
Pines

50

Kyburz

50

Placerville

ELDORADO
NATIONAL
FOREST

49

South Tahoe

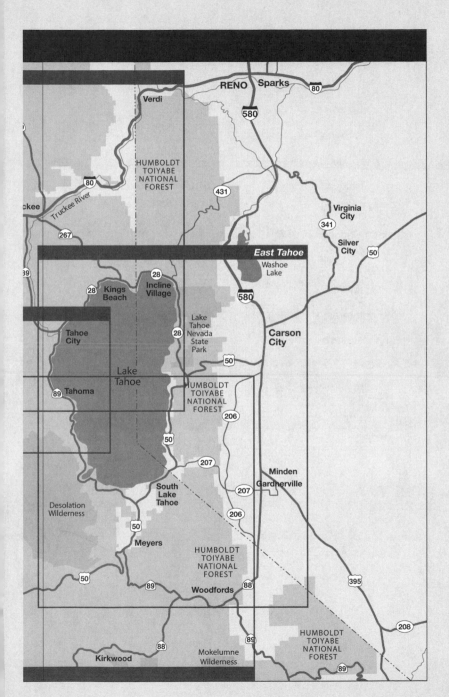

Map Legend

Trail	————————	Peak	▲
Other Trail	------------------------	River/Stream	～～～
Freeway	═══════════	Seasonal Stream	—·—·—·—
Road	————————		
Railroad	+—+—+—+—+—+	Body of Water	
Dirt Road	===================	Marsh/Swamp	⸈ ⸈ ⸈
Trailhead Parking	P	Park/Forest	
Gate	•—◦	Wilderness	
Start/Finish	🚶	Picnic Area	🛆
Point of Interest	■	Campground	△
Restrooms	♦♦	Lookout	⌖
Power Line	•—•—•—•		N
Building	🏠	North Arrow	🧭
Viewpoint	ᙢ		

Contents

CHAPTER 4

East Tahoe

Using Top Trails™

Organization of Top Trails

Top Trails is designed so you can find the perfect trail and make every outing a success and a pleasure. With this guide it's a snap to find the right trail, whether you're planning a major hike or just a sociable stroll with friends.

The Region

At the very front of this guide, the Lake Tahoe Trail Features Table (pages iv–vii) lists every trail covered in this guide, along with attributes for each trail.

The Lake Tahoe Overview Map (pages viii–ix) provides a geographic overview of the Lake Tahoe region and shows the areas covered by each chapter. A quick reading of the regional map and the trail features table gives you a quick overview of the entire region covered by the guide.

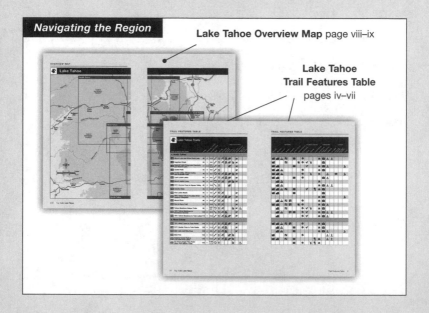

Navigating the Region

Lake Tahoe Overview Map page viii–ix

Lake Tahoe Trail Features Table pages iv–vii

The Areas

The region covered in this book is divided into areas, with each chapter corresponding to one area in the region. Each area chapter starts with information to help you choose and enjoy a trail every time out. Use the table of contents or the regional map to identify an area of interest, and then turn to the area chapter to find the following information:

- An overview of the area's parks and trails
- An area map showing all trail locations
- A trail features table providing trail-by-trail details
- Trail summaries highlighting each trail's special features

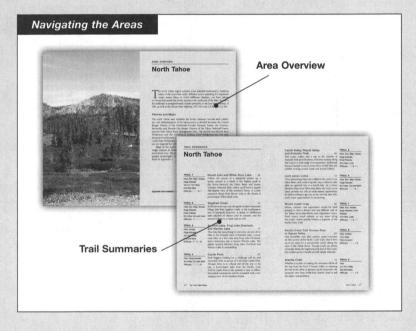

The Trails

The basic building block of the Top Trails guide is the trail entry. Each one is arranged to make finding and following the trail as simple as possible, with all pertinent information presented in this easy-to-follow format:

- A detailed trail map
- Trail descriptions covering difficulty, length, and other essential data
- A written trail description
- Trail milestones providing easy-to-follow, turn-by-turn trail directions

Some trail descriptions offer additional information:

- An elevation profile
- Trail options
- Trail highlights

In the margins of the trail entries, keep your eyes open for graphic icons that signal features mentioned in the text.

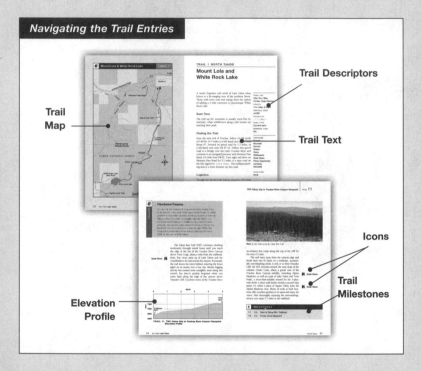

Choosing a Trail

Top Trails provides several different ways of choosing a trail, using easy-to-read tables and maps.

Location

If you know in general where you want to go, Top Trails makes it easy to find the right trail in the right place. Each chapter begins with a large-scale map showing the starting point of every trail in that area.

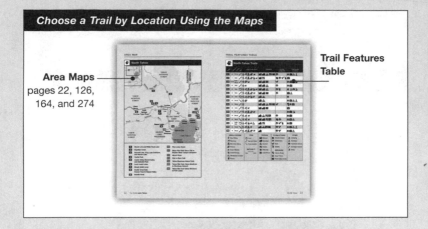

Choose a Trail by Location Using the Maps

Area Maps
pages 22, 126,
164, and 274

Trail Features
Table

Features

This guide describes the top trails of the Lake Tahoe region. Each trail has been chosen because it offers one or more features that make it interesting. Using the trail descriptors, summaries, and tables, you can quickly examine all the trails to find out what features they offer, or seek a particular feature among the list of trails.

Best Time

Time of year and current conditions can be important factors in selecting the best trail. For example, an exposed grassland trail may be a riot of color in early spring but an oven-baked taste of hell in midsummer. Other trails may be cool and shady all year. Where relevant, Top Trails identifies the best and worst conditions for the trails you plan to hike.

Difficulty

Each trail has an overall difficulty rating on a scale of 1–5, which takes into consideration length, elevation change, exposure, trail quality, and more to create one (admittedly subjective) rating.

The difficulty ratings assume that you are an able-bodied adult in reasonably good shape using the trail for hiking. The ratings also assume normal weather conditions—clear and dry.

Readers should make an honest assessment of their own abilities and adjust time estimates accordingly. Also, rain, snow, heat, mud, and poor visibility can all affect the pace on even the easiest of trails.

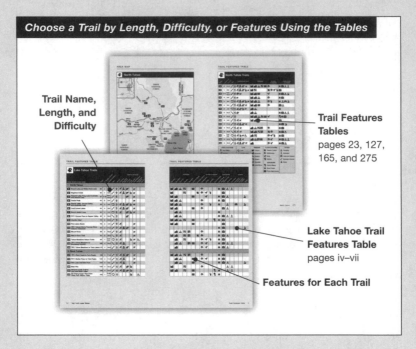

Choose a Trail by Length, Difficulty, or Features Using the Tables

Trail Name, Length, and Difficulty

Trail Features Tables
pages 23, 127, 165, and 275

Lake Tahoe Trail Features Table
pages iv–vii

Features for Each Trail

Vertical Feet

When gauging the difficulty of a trail, hikers and bikers often underestimate elevation change. Vertical feet accounts for all elevation change, not simply the difference between the highest and lowest points, so that rolling terrain with lots of up and down will be identifiable.

For routes that begin and end at the same spot—that is, a loop or out-and-back—the vertical gain exactly matches the vertical descent. With a point-to-point route, the vertical gain and loss will most likely differ, and both figures are provided in the text.

The more strenuous routes have an elevation profile, an easy means for visualizing the topography of a route. These profiles graphically depict the elevation throughout the length of the trail.

Top Trails Difficulty Ratings

1. A short trail, generally level, that can be completed in 1 hour or less.

2. A route of 1–3 miles, with some up and down, that can be completed in 1–2 hours.

3. A longer route, up to 5 miles, with uphill and/or downhill sections.

4. A long or steep route, perhaps more than 5 miles or climbs of more than 1,000 vertical feet.

5. The most severe, both long and steep, more than 5 miles long with climbs of more than 1,000 vertical feet.

Surface Type

Each trail entry provides information about the surface of the trail. This is useful in determining what type of footwear or bicycle is appropriate. Surface type should also be considered when checking the weather—on a rainy day a dirt surface can be a muddy slog; an asphalt surface might be a better choice (though asphalt can be slick when wet).

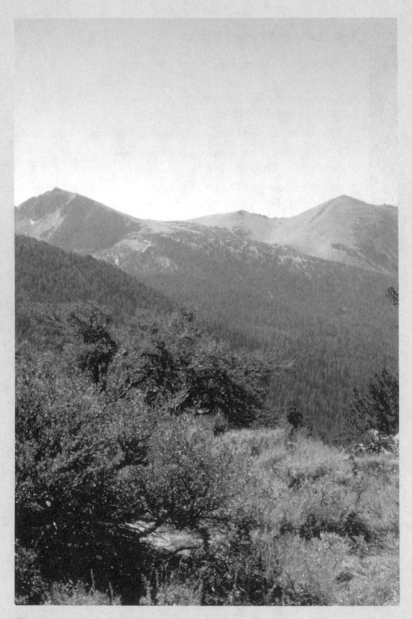

View south *toward Freel and Jobs Peaks (Trail 49)*

Introduction
to Lake Tahoe

T all mountains covered with a thick blanket of conifers surround the breathtakingly blue lake, creating a stunning, alplike setting, which is famous around the globe. Whether you plumb the depths of Lake Tahoe, climb to the summit of the highest peak, or journey somewhere in-between, the Tahoe Basin provides many opportunities to appreciate the grandeur of one of the West's most priceless treasures.

Geography and Topography

The Lake Tahoe Basin presents diverse topography that receives adoration from a devoted tourist base. At an elevation of 6,229 feet, Tahoe is the highest lake of its size in the United States and, with a depth of 1,645 feet (measured near Crystal Bay), is the third deepest lake in North America and the 10th deepest lake in the world. The 22-mile-long and 12-mile-wide lake has a 71-mile-long shoreline, with 42 of those scenic miles belonging to California and the remaining 29 owned by Nevada. Lake Tahoe is perhaps best known for the crystal clarity of its waters, which allows visibility of up to 75 feet below the surface. Sixty-three streams flow into Lake Tahoe, but only one, the Truckee River, flows out of the lake, reaching its terminus in the Great Basin, at Pyramid Lake.

Geologists speculate that the landform that would ultimately become the Tahoe Basin we know today was once beneath a shallow ancient sea in the supercontinent of Pangaea. The North American Continental Plate eventually broke away from Pangaea and headed west, colliding into the Pacific Ocean Plate, which was drifting east. Extreme pressure and heat were created as the North American Plate rose above the Pacific Plate, producing molten rock that slowly solidified beneath the sedimentary surface into granitic rocks, which were later exposed through faulting.

Faulting fractures in the earth's crust allowed blocks of land to rise and fall, pushing the primarily plutonic rocks of the Sierra Nevada up from the ancient seabed. Two principal faults evolved in the Tahoe area, which produced uplifts that became the main Sierra Crest to the west and the Carson

Range to the east. In between, the down-thrown fault block formed the deep V-shaped valley of the Tahoe Basin.

A lake began to form at the lowest, southern end of the basin, fed by precipitation and creeks draining the surrounding mountains. The level of the lake rose steadily, until an outlet for the river draining the lake was reached to the north, near the current town of Truckee. Later, a significant lava flow from Mount Pluto, site of the Northstar California Resort, dammed the outlet and caused the lake to rise again. Eventually the river was able to cut a new outlet through the volcanic rock, near the present-day Tahoe City. The highest level Lake Tahoe ever reached was an estimated 600 to 800 feet above the current level. Additional volcanic activity occurred at both the south end of the basin, around Carson Pass, and the north end of the basin, near Donner Pass.

Though a regional ice sheet was absent, in theory the last ice age put the finishing touches on the Tahoe Basin. Separate rivers of ice followed some of the existing V-shaped stream channels, carving them into classic U-shaped canyons. Glacial action scoured several of the canyons on the west side of the basin, uncovering the classic granite bedrock associated with the Sierra Nevada today. In the process, some of the area's most picturesque lakes were formed, including Donner, Cascade, Fallen Leaf, and Echo Lakes, as well as scenic Emerald Bay on Tahoe's southwest shore. Because the Sierra Crest creates a rain shadow effect, which limits the amount of precipitation, minimal glaciation occurred from the Carson Range to the east. Without the glacial scouring on the west side of the Tahoe Basin, the topography of the Carson Range is primarily volcanic soils rather than the classic Sierra granite bedrock. While the west side of the Tahoe Basin is sprinkled with an abundance of tarns, lakes, and ponds, the east side is nearly devoid of such features. Additional glacial activity influenced the area when ice dams formed across the Truckee River canyon and broke several times, producing floods that further shaped the canyon, depositing debris downstream as far away as present-day Reno.

Flora

Because the area ranges in elevation from 6,229 feet at lake level to 10,881 feet at the summit of Freel Peak, you can expect to encounter a wide range of flora on trails within the Tahoe Basin. The mountains and hills surrounding the beautiful shoreline of Lake Tahoe are carpeted with conifers. Though it's hard to believe at first glance, these trees belong almost exclusively to a second-growth forest, as the basin was nearly denuded to provide timber and fuel for Virginia City and the surrounding mines during the heyday of the

Comstock Lode. Though the varied vegetation defies strict classification, the following zones provide a general overview of Tahoe's flora.

The upper montane zone, the largest zone in the basin and containing the widest variety of plant types, runs from lake level to about 8,000 feet. The upper montane zone can be grouped into six distinct divisions. Up to around 7,000 feet, the white fir forest is named for the dominant member of a mixed forest, which also includes incense cedar, sugar pine, Jeffrey pine, and ponderosa pine, as well as red fir at the upper limits. Preferring a moist habitat, the white fir forest can form dense stands with little ground cover, or more open stands allowing deciduous trees and shrubs to thrive, including quaking aspen, willow, maple, currant, gooseberry, thimbleberry, and honeysuckle. Above the white fir forest, the red fir forest extends to about 8,500 feet. Unlike the white fir forest, red fir is found in exclusive stands, usually on cool northern or eastern exposures. The red fir forest is generally dense, allowing very little ground cover, which when present is composed primarily of shade-loving flowers and plants. The Jeffrey pine forest occupies drier slopes than those preferred by the white and red fir forests. Spanning elevations from lake level to approximately 8,000 feet, open Jeffrey pine forests intermix in the lower realms with sugar pine, ponderosa pine, white fir, and incense cedar. Those conifers are replaced by western white pine, ponderosa pine, and red fir toward the upper limits.

On southern exposures, light stands of Jeffrey pine forest oftentimes intermix with Sierra juniper or with open areas of montane chaparral. The drought-tolerant montane chaparral community spans elevations across the spectrum of the upper montane zone into the subalpine zone, typically occupying dry slopes with a southern exposure. This community incorporates several common shrubs, including huckleberry oak, tobacco brush, rabbitbrush, manzanita, chinquapin, and sagebrush. Along the eastern fringe of the Carson Range, mountain mahogany and juniper trees may dot the slopes of the montane chaparral community. Areas of sufficient groundwater produce the montane meadow community. Similar to the montane chaparral community, montane meadows span the realm of the upper montane zone into the subalpine zone. The wetter environment allows grasses, rushes, and sedges to thrive, along with several species of water-loving wildflowers. The last of the five classifications within the upper montane zone is the riparian community. With the additional moisture provided by perennial streams, lush foliage along the banks includes deciduous trees and shrubs such as aspen, cottonwood, willow, alder, creek dogwood, and mountain ash. Smaller plants and colorful wildflowers are also common in creek-side environments.

Above the upper montane zone, the subalpine zone begins around 8,000 feet and continues upward to timberline, which, depending on a number of variables, starts anywhere from 9,000 to 10,000 feet in the Tahoe Sierra. With characteristically poor soils and a harsh climate, where snow covers the ground for nine months of the year, the prolific forests below give way to isolated stands of conifers and the open terrain of meadows and talus slides. Red firs, lodgepole pines, and junipers may extend into this zone in some areas, with lodgepole pines often rimming the shoreline of subalpine lakes. Despite the sporadic appearance of these trees from the lower realm, the two conifer species most closely associated with the subalpine zone are mountain hemlock and whitebark pine. Nearing timberline, dwarfed and wind-battered whitebark pines become the only conifers able to survive the conditions of this harsh environment. Shrubs and plants in this zone also take on a diminished stature, hugging the ground in order to eke out an existence. Common plants include heathers and laurels. Where seeps and rivulets provide moist soils, a short-lived but stunning display of colorful wildflowers delights passersby. Rock outcrops may provide equally delight-ful displays of plants and flowers.

Above timberline, at the extreme upper elevations of the Tahoe Basin, is the alpine zone. Though there is some debate among botanists as to whether the Tahoe area has a well-defined alpine zone, only the backcountry traveler who reaches the summit of some of the basin's highest peaks will be able to observe the area in question. The vegetation within this zone appears to be a combination of tundra species from the north and desert species from the east. Whatever their origin, these plants are generally compact, low-growing perennials that grow rapidly and flower briefly, with most of their growth occurring belowground. Low-growing shrubs, such as low sagebrush and short-stemmed stenotus, share the extreme conditions and poor soils of the

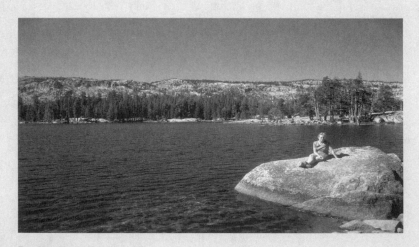

Dardanelles Lake *(Trail 38)*

alpine region with an assortment of wildflowers. The uppermost slopes of Mount Rose and Freel Peak provide some of the best opportunities in the Tahoe Sierra to experience the flora of the alpine zone.

Fauna

Along with a wide variety of plants, the Lake Tahoe Basin is home to a varied community of fauna. While traveling the trails around Lake Tahoe, with alert eyes you may be able to spot several different species of animals.

The largest mammal in the region is the omnivorous black bear, which ranges in color from black to cinnamon. Some members of Tahoe's black bear population, particularly near developed communities on the west shore, have become quite pesky in seeking food from garbage cans, dumpsters, and campgrounds. However, most bears you might see in the backcountry remain timid and are wary of human encounters. Though bears here are not nearly the nuisance that bears are in the backcountry of Yosemite, Kings Canyon, or Sequoia National Parks, backpackers should still obey basic bear safety guidelines (see below).

More likely to be seen along the trail than a bear in the Tahoe Sierra is the mule deer, so named for its floppy ears. Mule deer prefer varied terrain with an ample food supply, mainly leaves from trees and shrubs, along with grasses, sedges, and other herbs. Watch for mule deer around dusk in grassy meadows, or during the day in open forest where browse is plentiful. Deer herds in the Tahoe Basin are migratory, retreating in winter either west to the foothills or east to the Carson Valley. Since the extinction of the grizzly

 Bear Safety Guidelines

CAUTION: WILDLIFE

- Don't leave your pack unattended on the trail.
- Keep all food, trash, or scented items in a bear-proof canister or safely hung from a tree.
- Pack out all trash.
- Don't allow bears to approach your food—make noise, wave your arms, throw rocks. Be bold, but keep a safe distance and use good judgment.
- If a bear gets into your food, you are responsible for cleaning up the mess.
- Never attempt to retrieve food from a bear.
- Never approach a bear, especially a cub.
- Report any incidents to the appropriate authority.

bear and wolf from the Sierra, the mule deer's only natural predator is the mountain lion.

Though present in the greater Tahoe area, mountain lions, also known as cougars, are rarely seen by humans. Ranging in length from 6.5 to 8 feet and weighing as much as 200 pounds, mountain lions are primarily nocturnal, patrolling a vast range. Though mule deer are their principal food source, mountain lions will stalk smaller mammals as well. At an average weight of 20 pounds, the bobcat is the mountain lion's smaller cousin. Also nocturnal and equally reclusive, bobcats prefer a diet of rodents. You're much more likely to hear their blood-curdling scream during the night than see bobcats in the wild.

The highly adaptable coyote is often seen loping across the meadows and through the woodlands of Lake Tahoe. From backcountry campsites spread around the Tahoe Basin, backpackers frequently hear the coyote's nighttime chorus of howls and yelps. Though many area residents are familiar with the coyote, they fail to realize that it is omnivorous, preferring a diet of small rodents but also dining on berries and plants when such prey is unavailable.

Other common, medium-sized mammals of Lake Tahoe include martens, marmots, raccoons, porcupines, red foxes, weasels, and badgers. Hikers frequently see Douglas squirrels, California ground squirrels, golden-mantled ground squirrels, western gray squirrels, western flying squirrels, and chipmunks. Smaller rodents include pikas, voles, shrews, mice, moles, and pocket gophers.

At dusk, backpackers camped around one of Tahoe's backcountry lakes are almost guaranteed a visit from a handful of bats searching the skies for the evening's first course of insects. Midsummer visitors will be comforted to know that large helpings of mosquitoes are on the bats' menu.

The skies above the Lake Tahoe Basin are home to hundreds of bird species. While hiking around the shore of Lake Tahoe or the banks of rivers and creeks, keep your eyes peeled for bald eagles and ospreys, though they are not particularly common. Red-tailed hawks are the raptors more frequently seen patrolling the skies. Great horned owls are primarily nocturnal but may be seen napping on a tree limb during the day. A walk along Tahoe's trails without seeing a Clark's nutcracker, mountain chickadee, or Steller's jay is hard to imagine. Numerous songbirds fly around the Tahoe Basin, but a fine treat would be the sighting of a mountain bluebird flitting about a subalpine meadow or perched on the branch of a young lodgepole pine near the edge.

Amphibians and reptiles are common residents of the area. The most frequently seen species include the Pacific tree frog, the western fence lizard, and the common garter snake. Though possible, encountering a western rattlesnake in the Lake Tahoe Basin is extremely unlikely.

Insects are abundant members of the Lake Tahoe community. Unfortunately, the mosquito gains the most attention. Thankfully, depending on elevation and the rate at which the previous winter's snowpack melts, the peak of the mosquito season lasts for just a few weeks in the backcountry, usually through the last weeks of July into the first week of August.

The lakes and streams of the Tahoe Basin teem with fish, where anglers can ply their craft in search of brook, brown, cutthroat, and rainbow trout. Along with these trout, Lake Tahoe itself is home to a couple of introduced species: Mackinaw, also known as lake trout, and Kokanee salmon. Biologists theorize that Mackinaws in Lake Tahoe may reach a weight as high as 50 pounds, but the record catch so far is 37 pounds, 6 ounces. Landlocked cousins of the sockeye salmon, Kokanee salmon were introduced to Lake Tahoe in 1944. The Taylor Creek Stream Profile Chamber at the Taylor Creek Visitor Center (Trail 30) provides an excellent opportunity for viewing the annual spawning migration of the Kokanee each autumn, usually coinciding with the locally renowned Kokanee Festival, held the first week of October.

When to Go

Though Lake Tahoe is considered a year-round recreation destination, those wishing to hike snow-free trails will have to wait until the summer hiking season, when the previous winter's snowpack has melted and the customarily pleasant weather has settled into the region. Trails begin to shed their winter mantle at lake level as early as mid- to late April, with the snow line progressively receding up the mountainside until the highest elevations are clear, usually no later than mid-July. The wildflower bloom generally begins in earnest a couple of weeks after snowmelt, which varies, depending on such factors as elevation, exposure, and temperature.

On par with many locations in the desert Southwest, the Lake Tahoe Basin has a 93% probability of sunshine for any day from June through August. However, unlike the desert Southwest, mild summer temperatures rarely exceed 80°F. With the moderating influences of both the lake's 193-square-mile surface area and the dense forests surrounding the lake, nighttime temperatures stay mild during the summer months as well, with lows ranging from the high 30s in June to the low 40s in July and August. Precipitation during the summer is generally light at lake level, with averages of 0.69 inch for June, 0.26 inch for July, and 0.31 inch for August. Most of that falls during thunderstorms, which can be intense at higher elevations in the mountains. Unlike the Rocky Mountains, the Tahoe Sierra may experience summers of little or no thunderstorms, or a run of days when they're fairly frequent. Hikers should always be prepared for an afternoon cloudburst and to beat a hasty retreat from higher elevations when lightning is threatening.

Warm, dry weather often lingers through the waning days of summer and occasionally through the end of September and into October. The Tahoe area is usually blessed during autumn, when temperatures are cooler but still pleasant enough for hiking. In October, when fall color adorns the meadows and stream canyons of the Tahoe Basin, the average high temperature is 57°F and, though the average monthly precipitation climbs to 1.9 inches, there is still an 84% chance of having a sunny day. Usually in November a Pacific storm brings the first significant snowfall to the mountains, encouraging hikers to trade in their boots for skis or snowshoes.

Because Lake Tahoe is such a popular summer destination, many of the trails are heavily used during the height of the tourist season. Weekends between Memorial Day and Labor Day can be particularly crowded, especially on the southwest side of the lake. When contemplating a trip for June, July, or August, plan on hiking during the week. If a weekday adventure is out of the question, try to arrive early on the weekends to secure a parking spot and to beat the hordes up the trail. Desolation Wilderness has long been one of the most visited wilderness areas in the United States, resulting in quotas and fees for overnight users. Though the number of day hikers is not limited, trailhead registration is required for entry into the wilderness. While Lake Tahoe can be a bit of a human zoo during the summer at some localities, a good percentage of the backcountry sees light to moderate use.

Fall provides some of the finest trail experiences of the year. After Labor Day weekend the Tahoe area sees a diminishing number of tourists, a trend that continues as the days progress, until ski season begins. With good weather the norm and fewer people competing for space on the trail, hikers can experience the grandeur of the Tahoe backcountry in uncrowded fashion.

Trail Selection

Several criteria were used to arrange this assortment of Tahoe's 50 best trails. Only the premier hikes, runs, and rides were included, based on beautiful scenery, ease of access, quality of trail, and diversity of experience. Some of the trails selected are highly popular, while others may see infrequent use. Anyone fortunate enough to complete all the trips in this guide would have a comprehensive appreciation for the natural beauty of one of the West's most scenic recreational havens.

About 70% of the trails included in this guide are classified as out-and-back trips, requiring you to retrace your steps back to a trailhead. The remaining percentage is roughly distributed between point-to-point, loop, and partial-loop trips.

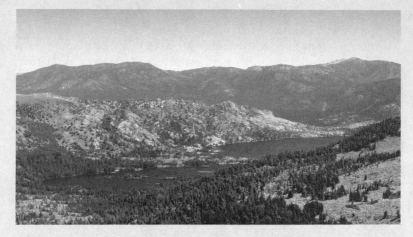

Echo Lakes *(Trail 34)*

Key Features

Top Trails books contain information about features for each trail. Though primarily a mountainous region, the Lake Tahoe Basin has such outstanding diversity that it offers at least a little of each feature, including sandy beaches. Lakes, streams, and waterfalls occur in abundance, as do high summits with spectacular vistas and rugged canyons. A plethora of verdant meadows are graced with scenic wildflower displays, and numerous aspen groves provide plenty of autumn color. All these features combine to make Lake Tahoe and the surrounding topography a photographer's paradise. About the only feature that suffers in the Lake Tahoe region is solitude, due in some part to the abundance of these other attributes.

Multiple Uses

All the trails in this guide are suitable for hiking, with the exception of the Flume Trail (Trail 46). Even though hikers are permitted to use it, the Flume Trail is so popular with mountain bikers that hikers should yield their rights to the two-wheeled crowd. Though all the trails are equally legal for runners, some have been determined impractical for such use.

Lake Tahoe has become one of the West's premier meccas for mountain bikers. Mountain biking is not permitted on the Pacific Crest Trail or in the wilderness areas around Lake Tahoe, which currently include Mount Rose, Granite Chief, Desolation, and Mokelumne Wildernesses. If two proposed wilderness areas become reality, this ban may extend to areas around Castle Peak and Meiss Meadows. Other trails—though they may be administratively classified as multiuse trails—have been excluded from prospective use by mountain bikes because of unsuitable terrain or conditions.

Equestrians will find plenty of trails within the Lake Tahoe Basin to ride. A handful of trails have been restricted from equestrian use by governmental agencies, primarily for environmental concerns or a high probability of conflict between horses and humans. Others are not recommended for horses because of unsuitable terrain.

Trail Safety

Elevations in the Lake Tahoe Basin vary from 6,229 feet at lake level to 10,881 feet at the summit of Freel Peak. Though these elevations are not considered extreme by mountaineering standards, people living near sea level who recreate at the higher elevations may experience symptoms of altitude sickness. These include headache, fatigue, loss of appetite, shortness of breath, nausea, vomiting, drowsiness, dizziness, memory loss, and loss of mental acuity. Untreated, altitude sickness can lead to acute mountain sickness, which is more serious and requires immediate medical attention.

To avoid altitude sickness, acclimatize slowly, drink plenty of fluids, and eat a diet high in carbohydrates prior to your trip. A rapid descent generally alleviates any symptoms if they develop. A severe case of altitude sickness is unlikely, though not impossible, at elevations around the lake.

Less atmosphere to filter the sun's rays at higher altitudes increases the risks of exposure to the sun. Wear an appropriate sunblock on exposed areas, and reapply as necessary. Sunglasses will protect the eyes, which is especially important in areas where the sun reflects off snowfields or the granite bedrock that is prevalent on the west side of the basin.

Dehydration is another potential hazard while recreating in the backcountry of Lake Tahoe. Carry and drink plenty of fluids while on the trail. Any water gathered from streams or lakes should be filtered or treated. Some of the trails in the Tahoe area, particularly in the Carson Range, have long, waterless stretches, so plan on packing extra water in those areas.

Though the weather in the mountains around Lake Tahoe is predictably fair, conditions can change rapidly at any time. Be sure to pack appropriate clothing to endure any change in the weather. Even if the day is fair, temperatures can be radically different at lake level than at the summit of a windswept peak like Mount Tallac or Freel Peak. Dousing thunderstorms can leave the ill prepared wet, cold, and potentially hypothermic; snowfall has occurred at Lake Tahoe during every month of the year.

Mosquitoes can be a major irritant for recreationists during midsummer, when long pants, long-sleeved shirts, and mosquito netting are good apparel choices. Application and reapplication of an insect repellent with plenty of

DEET should keep the winged pests at bay. Clothing manufacturers have developed lines of pants, shirts, scarves, and hats that have insect repellent infused into the fabrics, and products are also available to wash this protection into your clothes at home. Such measures are a good deterrent against ticks as well, though they are generally much less of a nuisance. There is a remote possibility, however, that a tick could infect you with Lyme disease or Rocky Mountain spotted fever. Inspect your body for bites at least once a day and check your clothes for any unwanted travelers. If you are bitten by a tick, firmly grasp the pest with a pair of tweezers and use gentle traction for its removal, making sure that the head is not left behind. After successful removal of the entire tick, wash the area thoroughly with antibacterial soap and water and apply an antibiotic ointment. Consult a physician if flulike symptoms, headache, rash, joint pain, or fever develop.

Camping and Permits

Plenty of camping opportunities exist around the greater Lake Tahoe area. The hard part may be securing a spot, as many of the campgrounds are extremely popular during the summer months, especially on weekends. Reservations are recommended between Memorial Day weekend and Labor Day weekend. The U.S. Forest Service manages the bulk of public campgrounds in the greater Lake Tahoe area. California State Parks and Nevada State Parks manage several excellent campgrounds as well. South Lake Tahoe and Tahoe City each offer a public campground. In addition, there are a number of private campgrounds, including popular Camp Richardson, on the southwest shore.

Desolation Wilderness is the one area in the Tahoe Basin that requires day hikers to secure a permit. Self-registration is available at most trailheads. Otherwise, permits can be obtained from the Lake Tahoe Visitor Center near Fallen Leaf Lake.

Wilderness permits are required for backpackers entering Desolation Wilderness or Mokelumne Wilderness. More specific information on these permits is provided in the chapter on trails in South Tahoe. Backpackers using the Pacific Crest Trail or Tahoe Rim Trail must use portable gas stoves (no campfires) and obtain a campfire permit for their use. At the time of research, wilderness permits were not required for overnight use of Granite Chief Wilderness or Mount Rose Wilderness.

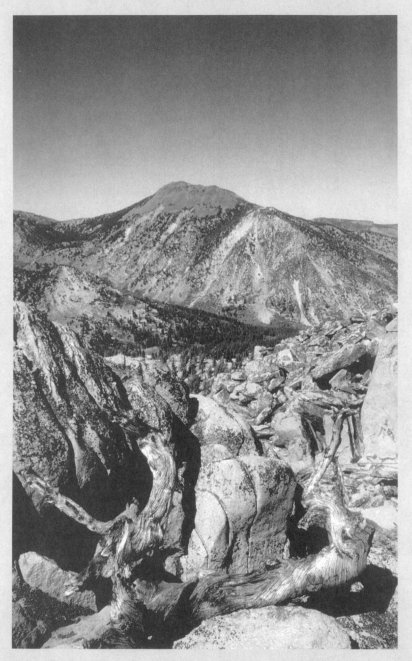

Mount Rose (*Trail 12*)

On the Trail

Every outing should begin with proper preparation. Even the easiest trail can turn up unexpected surprises. People seldom think about getting lost or suffering an injury, but unexpected things can and do happen. A few minutes' worth of simple precautions can make the difference between a marvelous and a miserable outcome—or merely a good story to tell afterward.

Use the Top Trails ratings and descriptions to determine if a particular trail is a good match with your fitness and energy level, given current conditions and time of year.

Have a Plan

Choose Wisely The first step to enjoying any trail is to match the trail to your abilities. It's no use overestimating your experience or fitness—know your abilities and limitations, and use the Top Trails difficulty rating that accompanies each trail.

Leave Word About Your Plans The most basic of precautions is leaving word of your intentions with family or friends. Many people will hike the backcountry their entire lives without ever relying on this safety net, but establishing this simple habit is free insurance.

It's best to leave specific information—location, trail name, intended time of travel—with a responsible person. If there is a registration process, make use of it. If there is a ranger station or park office, check in.

Review the Route Before embarking on any trail, be sure to read the entire description and study the map. It isn't necessary to memorize every detail,

Prepare and Plan

- Know your abilities and your limitations.
- Leave word about your plans with family or friends.
- Know the area and the route.

13

but it is worthwhile to have a clear mental picture of the trail and the general area. If the trail and terrain are complex, augment the trail guide with a topographic map. Park maps, as well as current weather and trail condition information, are often available from local ranger stations and at trailheads.

Carry the Essentials

Proper preparation for any type of trail use includes gathering the essential items to carry. Your checklist may vary according to choice of trails and daily conditions.

Clothing If the weather is good, then light, comfortable clothing is the obvious choice. It's easy to believe that very little spare clothing is needed, but a prepared hiker has something tucked away for any emergency from a surprise shower to an unexpected overnight in a remote area.

Clothing includes proper footwear, essential for hiking and running trails. As a trail becomes more demanding, you will need footwear that performs. Running shoes are fine for many trails. If you will be carrying substantial weight or encountering sustained rugged terrain, step up to hiking boots and synthetic or wool-blend (not cotton) socks specifically designed for hiking.

In hot, sunny weather, proper clothing includes a hat, sunglasses, long-sleeved shirt, and sunscreen. In cooler weather, particularly when it's wet, carry waterproof outer garments and quick-drying undergarments (avoid cotton). As a general rule, whatever the conditions, bring layers that can be combined or removed to provide comfort and protection from the elements in a wide variety of conditions.

Water Never embark on a trail without carrying water. For most outings, you should plan to carry sufficient water to last you and your entire party the entire hike (including the return trip). At all times, particularly in warm weather, adequate water is of key importance. Experts recommend at least 2 quarts of water per person per day, and when hiking in heat 1 gallon or more may be more appropriate. At the extreme, dehydration can be life threatening. More commonly, inadequate water brings on fatigue and muscle aches.

If it's necessary to make use of trailside water, you should filter or chemically treat it. You should regard all untreated water sources as being contaminated with bacteria, viruses, and fertilizers. There are three methods for treating water: boiling, chemical treatment, and filtering. Boiling is best but often impractical—it requires a heat source, a pot, and time. Chemical treatments, available in sporting goods and outdoor stores, handle some problems, including the troublesome *Giardia* parasite, but will not combat many human-made chemical pollutants. The most practical method is filtration, which removes *Giardia* and other contaminants and doesn't leave any unpleasant aftertaste.

One final admonishment: Be prepared for surprises. Water sources described in the text or on maps can change course or dry up completely. Never run your water bottle dry in expectation of the next source; fill up when water is available and always keep a little in reserve.

Food Though not as critical as water, food is energy and its importance should not be underestimated. Avoid foods that are hard to digest, such as candy bars and potato chips. Carry high-energy, fast-digesting foods, such as nutrition bars, dehydrated fruit, nuts, trail mix, and jerky. Bringing a little extra food is good protection against an outing that turns unexpectedly long, perhaps due to weather or losing your way.

Less Than Essential, But Useful Items

Map and Compass (and the Know-How to Use Them) Many trails don't require much navigation, meaning a map and compass aren't always as essential, but they can be useful. If the trail is remote or infrequently visited, a map and compass should be considered necessities.

A handheld GPS (Global Positioning System) receiver can also be a useful trail companion, but is really no substitute for a map and compass; knowing your longitude and latitude is not much help without a map.

Cell Phone Most parts of the country, even remote destinations, have some level of cellular coverage. In extreme circumstances, a cell phone can be a lifesaver, but don't depend on it; coverage is unpredictable and batteries fail. And be sure that the occasion warrants the phone call—a blister doesn't justify a call to search and rescue.

Gear Depending on the remoteness and rigor of the trail, there are many additional useful items to consider: pocketknife, flashlight, fire source (waterproof matches, light, or flint), and a first-aid kit.

Every member of your party should carry the appropriate essential items described above; groups often split up or get separated along the trail. Solo hikers should be even more disciplined about preparation and make a habit of carrying a little more gear than absolutely necessary. Traveling solo is inherently more risky. This isn't meant to discourage solo travel, simply to emphasize the need for extra preparation.

Trail Etiquette

The overriding rule on the trail is "Leave No Trace." Interest in visiting natural areas continues to increase, even as the quantity of unspoiled natural areas continues to shrink. These pressures make it ever more critical that we leave no trace of our visit.

Never Litter If you carried it in, it's easy enough to carry it out. Leave the trail in the same, if not better, condition than you find it. Try picking up any litter you encounter and packing it out—it's a great feeling! Pack a spare plastic bag to carry litter. Just picking up a few pieces of garbage makes a difference.

Stay on the Trail Paths have been created, sometimes over many years, for many purposes: to protect the surrounding natural areas, to avoid dangers, and to provide the best route. Leaving the trail can cause damage that takes years to undo. Never cut switchbacks. Shortcutting rarely saves energy or time, and it takes a terrible toll on the land, trampling plant life and hastening erosion. Moreover, safety and consideration intersect on the trail. It's hard to get truly lost if you stay on the trail.

Share the Trail The best trails attract many visitors and you should be prepared to share the trail with others. Do your part to minimize impact. Commonly accepted trail etiquette dictates that bike riders yield to both hikers and equestrians, hikers yield to horseback riders, downhill hikers yield to uphill hikers, and everyone stays to the right. Not everyone knows these rules of the road, so let common sense and good humor be the final guide.

Trail Etiquette

- Leave no trace. Never litter.
- Stay on the trail.
- Share the trail.
- Leave it there.

Leave It There Destruction or removal of plants and animals or historical, prehistoric, or geological items is certainly unethical and almost always illegal.

Getting Lost If you become lost on the trail, stay on the trail. Stop and take stock of the situation. In many cases, a few minutes of calm reflection will yield a solution. Consider all the clues available; use the sun to identify directions if you don't have a compass. If you determine that you are indeed lost, stay put. You are more likely to encounter other people if you stay in one place.

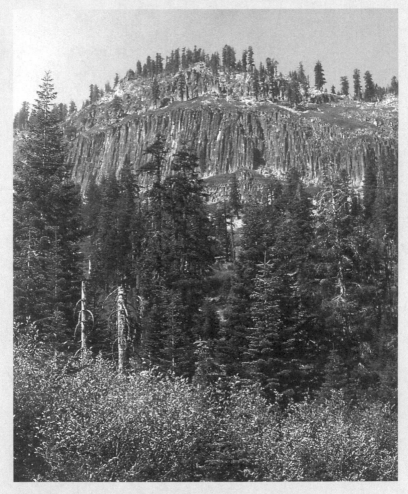

Cliffs in Powderhorn Canyon (*Trail 20*)

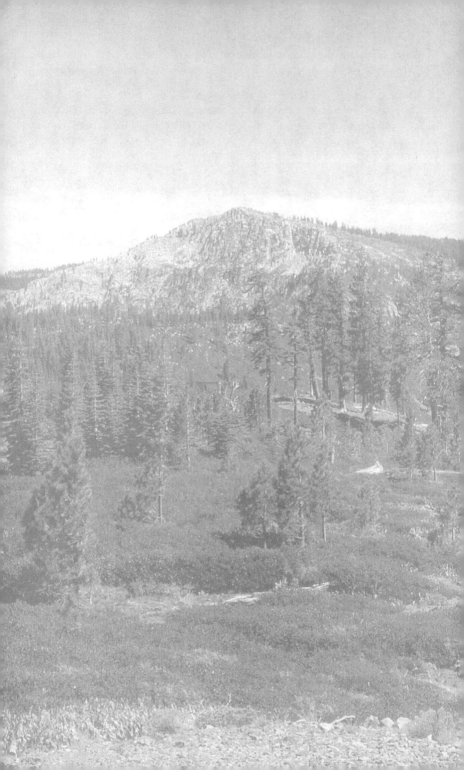

North Tahoe

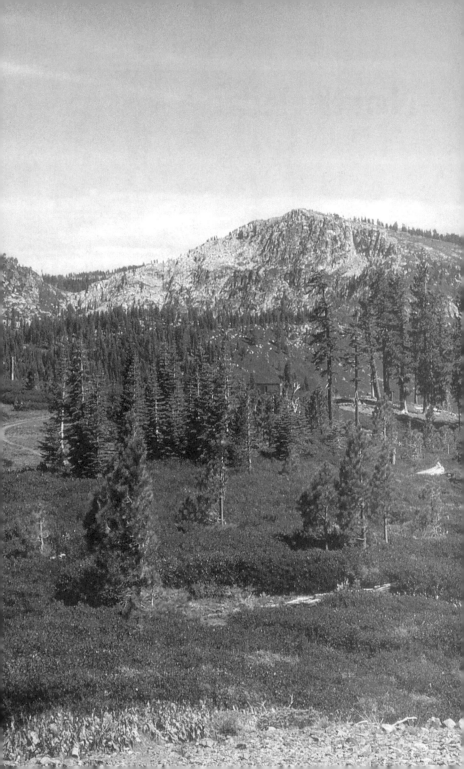

North Tahoe

T he north Tahoe region contains some splendid backcountry, boasting many of the area's best trails. Whether you're searching for expansive vistas, serene lakes, or vivid wildflower displays, you have plenty to choose from amid the diverse terrain at the north end of the lake. Access to the trailheads is straightforward, thanks primarily to the four-lane freeway of I-80, as well as the Mount Rose Highway (NV 431) and CA 89 and CA 267.

Permits and Maps

The north Tahoe area straddles the border between Nevada and California, and administration of the backcountry is divided between the Carson Ranger District of the Humboldt–Toiyabe National Forest; the Truckee, Sierraville, and Nevada City Ranger Districts of the Tahoe National Forest; and the Lake Tahoe Basin Management Unit. The 28,000-acre Mount Rose Wilderness and the 19,050-acre Granite Chief Wilderness are the only designated wilderness areas at the north end of the lake, but the proposed Castle Peak Wilderness would add another 18,000 acres. Currently, permits are not required for either day or overnight trips.

Maps of the north Tahoe region are available at U.S. Forest Service ranger stations in Nevada City, Grass Valley, Sierraville, Truckee, Sparks, and Carson City. The best maps for trail use are the USGS 7.5-minute topographic quadrangles. Specific maps for the trails covered in this section are listed in Appendix 4.

Opposite and overleaf: *Castle Peak (Trail 4)*

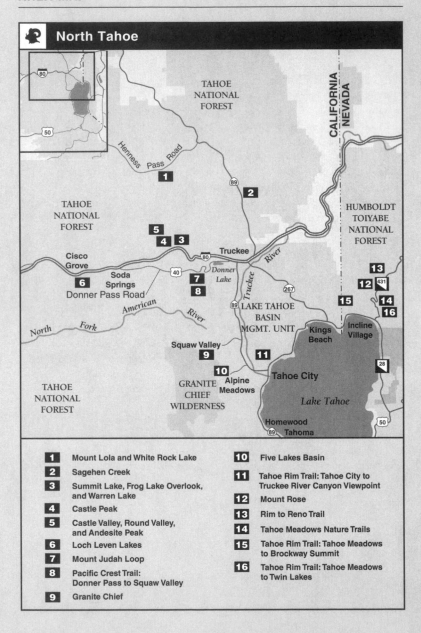

North Tahoe

TAHOE NATIONAL FOREST

CALIFORNIA
NEVADA

1

2

TAHOE NATIONAL FOREST

HUMBOLDT TOIYABE NATIONAL FOREST

5
4 **3**

Truckee

Cisco Grove

Soda Springs
Donner Pass Road

6

Donner Lake

7
8

13

12

15

14
16

American River

North Fork

Squaw Valley

9

LAKE TAHOE BASIN MGMT. UNIT

Kings Beach

Incline Village

10 Alpine Meadows

GRANITE CHIEF WILDERNESS

11

Tahoe City

Lake Tahoe

28

TAHOE NATIONAL FOREST

Homewood
Tahoma

50

1	Mount Lola and White Rock Lake	**10**	Five Lakes Basin
2	Sagehen Creek	**11**	Tahoe Rim Trail: Tahoe City to Truckee River Canyon Viewpoint
3	Summit Lake, Frog Lake Overlook, and Warren Lake	**12**	Mount Rose
4	Castle Peak	**13**	Rim to Reno Trail
5	Castle Valley, Round Valley, and Andesite Peak	**14**	Tahoe Meadows Nature Trails
6	Loch Leven Lakes	**15**	Tahoe Rim Trail: Tahoe Meadows to Brockway Summit
7	Mount Judah Loop	**16**	Tahoe Rim Trail: Tahoe Meadows to Twin Lakes
8	Pacific Crest Trail: Donner Pass to Squaw Valley		
9	Granite Chief		

North Tahoe Trails

TRAIL	DIFFICULTY	LENGTH	TYPE	USES & ACCESS	TERRAIN	FLORA & FAUNA	EXPOSURE & OTHER
1	4	14.4					
2	1	5.0					
3	1–5	4.0–15.0					
4	5	9.6					
5	3	9.6					
6	4	8.0					
7	3	4.6					
8	5	15.0					
9	5	10.2					
10	3	4.0					
11	4	11.4					
12	3	10.0					
13	5	18.0					
14	1	0.8–3.3					
15	5	19.5					
16	4	19.0					

USES & ACCESS
- Day Hiking
- Running
- Mountain Biking
- Horses
- Dogs Allowed
- Child-Friendly
- Wheelchair Access
- Permit

TYPE
- Loop
- Out-and-back
- Point-to-point

DIFFICULTY
- 1 2 3 4 5 +
  less   more

TERRAIN
- Canyon
- Mountain
- Summit
- Stream
- Waterfall
- Lake/Shore

FLORA & FAUNA
- Autumn Colors
- Wildflowers
- Birds
- Wildlife

EXPOSURE
- Cool & Shady
- Great Views
- Photo Opportunity

OTHER
- Camping
- Secluded
- Historical Interest
- Geologic Interest
- Steep

North Tahoe

Castle Valley, Round Valley, and Andesite Peak

.... 48

Two scenic valleys and a trip to the summit of Andesite Peak provide plenty of diverse scenery along this loop for a wide range of recreationists. Additional bonuses include a visit to rustic Peter Grubb Hut and wildlife viewing around Castle and Round Valleys.

TRAIL 5

Hike, Run, Bike, Horses,
Dogs Allowed,
Child Friendly
9.6 miles, Loop
Difficulty: 1 2 **3** 4 5

Loch Leven Lakes 54

Three picturesque lakes are cradled in the Loch Leven Lakes basin, and a mile-long side trip to Salmon Lake adds an optional visit to a fourth lake. At a lower elevation than most Tahoe-area lakes, the Loch Leven Lakes provide not only an early-season opportunity for hikers itching to get out on the trail but also relatively warm opportunities for swimming.

TRAIL 6

Hike, Run, Bike, Horses,
Dogs Allowed
8.0 miles, Out-and-back
Difficulty: 1 2 3 **4** 5

Mount Judah Loop 60

Hikers, runners, and equestrians would be hard pressed to find a shorter and less difficult trail in the Tahoe Sierra that affords such impressive views. Don't expect much solitude or any water along this route, which initially follows a segment of the Pacific Crest Trail.

TRAIL 7

Hike, Run, Horses,
Dogs Allowed, Child
Friendly
4.6 miles, Loop
Difficulty: 1 2 **3** 4 5

Pacific Crest Trail: Donner Pass to Squaw Valley 65

One incredible view after another awaits travelers on this section of the Pacific Crest Trail, which lives up to its name for a several-mile course along the crest of the Tahoe Sierra. Though you'll see plenty of people along the beginning and end of this route, the middle section should provide ample solitude.

TRAIL 8

Hike, Horses
15.0 miles,
Point-to-point
Difficulty: 1 2 3 4 **5**

Granite Chief 72

Whether you plan on making the strenuous climb all the way from the floor of Squaw Valley or enjoying the ride in the cable car partway up the mountain, the awesome view from 9,006-foot Granite Chief is still the same—extraordinary.

TRAIL 9

Hike
2.5–10.2 miles,
Out-and-back
Difficulty: 1 2 3 4 **5**

Tahoe Rim Trail: Tahoe Meadows to Brockway Summit 105

TRAIL 15

Hike, Run, Bike,
Dogs Allowed
19.5 miles,
Point-to-point
Difficulty: 1 2 3 4 **5**

Several miles of this section of the Tahoe Rim Trail cross south-facing volcanic slopes at or just below the crest of an exposed ridge. Here are some of the most panoramic Lake Tahoe views available anywhere in the basin. The 19.5-mile distance, combined with a lack of access from connecting trails, ensures that you'll have most of the trail to yourself, at least in the middle of the route.

Tahoe Rim Trail: Tahoe Meadows to Twin Lakes 115

TRAIL 16

Hike, Run, Horses,
Bike (even days only),
Dogs Allowed
19.0 miles,
Out-and-back
Difficulty: 1 2 3 **4** 5

After an initial climb from Tahoe Meadows, this part of the Tahoe Rim Trail closely follows the crest of the Carson Range, offering fine views of Lake Tahoe to the west and the Great Basin to the east. A number of connecting roads and trails present plenty of trip alternatives, especially for mountain bikers.

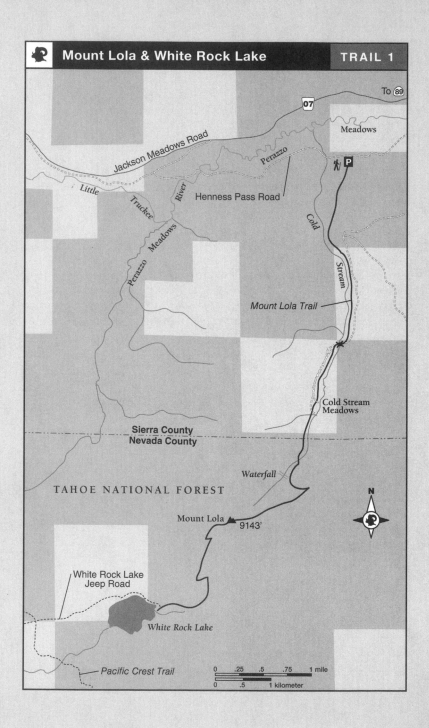

07

To **89**

Meadows

Jackson Meadows Road

Perazzo

Little

Henness Pass Road

Truckee

River

Perazzo Meadows

Cold

Stream

Mount Lola Trail

Cold Stream Meadows

Sierra County
Nevada County

Waterfall

TAHOE NATIONAL FOREST

Mount Lola ▲ 9143'

N

White Rock Lake
Jeep Road

White Rock Lake

Pacific Crest Trail

| 0 | .25 | .5 | .75 | 1 mile |
| 0 | | .5 | | 1 kilometer |

Mount Lola and White Rock Lake

A nearly forgotten trail north of Lake Tahoe takes hikers to a far-ranging view of the northern Sierra. Those with extra time and energy have the option of adding a 2-mile extension to picturesque White Rock Lake.

Best Time

The trail up the mountain is usually snow-free by mid-July, when wildflowers along Cold Stream are entering their peak.

Finding the Trail

Near the west end of Truckee, follow CA 89 north of I-80 for 14.5 miles to a left-hand turn onto Forest Route 07. Proceed on paved road for 1.5 miles, to a left-hand turn onto FR 07-10. Follow this gravel road to a bridge over the Little Truckee River and continue to an unsigned junction with Henness Pass Road, 0.6 mile from FR 07. Turn right and drive on Henness Pass Road for 3.1 miles to a spur road on the left, signed MT LOLA TRAIL. The trailhead parking area is a short distance up this road.

Logistics

Though the Mount Lola Trail is closed to all motor vehicles, a four-wheel-drive road closely parallels the trail through Cold Stream Valley. In addition, White Rock Lake is accessible to four-wheel-drive vehicles via a road on the west side of the lake.

TRAIL USE
Hike, Run, Bike,
Horses, Dogs Allowed
LENGTH
14.4 miles, 8 hours
VERTICAL FEET
±2,550
DIFFICULTY
– 1 2 3 **4 5** +
TRAIL TYPE
Out-and-back
SURFACE TYPE
Dirt

FEATURES
Canyon
Mountain
Summit
Stream
Shore
Wildflowers
Great Views
Photo Opportunity
Camping
Secluded

FACILITIES
None

At 9,143 feet, Mount Lola is the highest summit between the Tahoe Basin and Lassen Volcanic National Park.

Trail Description

▶1 Singletrack trail leads away from the trailhead on a moderate climb through mixed forest of western white pines, lodgepole pines, and white firs. At 0.6 mile, hop across a small seasonal stream lined with a tangle of alders and young aspens and continue the climb toward the mouth of Cold Stream Canyon. Where the singletrack trail merges with an old roadbed, you head upstream high above the level of the creek. Gaps in the mixed forest allow enough sunlight for an understory of tobacco brush, pine-mat manzanita, and currant. Farther up the canyon the trail eventually draws closer to Cold Stream before intersecting a well-traveled road, 2.2 miles from the trailhead.

Walk along the road to a substantial wood bridge that spans the stream, and soon encounter a fork in the road. Take the left-hand fork and head upstream a short way to the resumption of single-track trail on the left, which is unsigned but marked by a series of metal diamonds. Within a stone's throw of the road to the right and the creek to the left, you continue upstream on mildly graded trail beneath mixed forest until breaking out into the open at Cold Stream Meadows. Dotted with clumps of willow and carpeted with a variety of grasses and

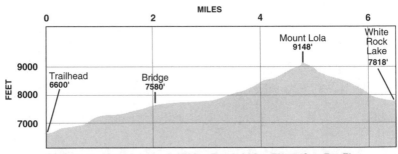

TRAIL 1   Mount Lola & White Rock Lake Elevation Profile

wildflowers, the meadow lends a pastoral feel to the surroundings. A spur road near the far end of the meadow leads to a campsite in a copse of trees that's sure to lure overnighters.

Just beyond the spur to the campsite, the route follows the main road briefly until singletrack trail resumes where the road bends sharply toward a crossing of Cold Stream. You proceed upstream for a while on mildly graded trail, hopping over a pair of tiny rivulets along the way. As the canyon narrows, the grade of the ascent increases and the trail draws nearer to the diminishing stream, crossing to the east bank at 3.8 miles from the trailhead.

Camping

You climb more steeply up the canyon after the creek crossing, reaching a faint use trail after 0.25 mile that soon leads to a view of a short waterfall, where the braided stream courses through moss-covered channels and tumbles picturesquely down a slanted rock face. Beyond the fall, the trail angles away from Cold Creek and ascends into the realm of mountain hemlocks. After a prominent switchback, the trees part enough to allow a glimpse of the upper slopes of Mount Lola and, as you follow the winding trail up the northeast ridge of the peak, other landmarks spring into view, including Independence

Stream

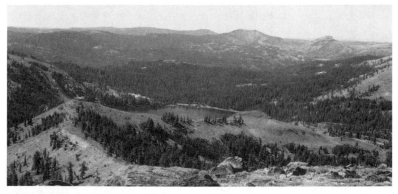

White Rock Lake *from Mount Lola*

Lake to the east and Castle Peak to the south. Reaching the summit, the incredible 360-degree view is ample reward for the toil of the ascent. ►2 Scores of peaks are visible from Mount Lola, including Lassen Peak, Sierra Buttes, Mount Rose, and Freel Peak. You'll also see verdant plains such as Sierra Valley and Martis Valley, and many bodies of water, such as Stampede, Boca, and Prosser Reservoirs. An old wooden sign reading MT. LOLA, ELEV. 9143 FT. marks the top, along with some low brick pillars, a few rock enclosures, and a metal army box holding the summit register. A short walk to the southern lip of the summit area reveals the shimmering surface of White Rock Lake, a mere 1.25 miles southwest of Mount Lola.

To reach White Rock Lake, weave your way down the trail on the southwest ridge of the volcanic mountain amid low-growing shrubs, scattered wildflowers, and a few stunted pines farther down the ridge. After a couple of switchbacks, you make a descending traverse across the head of a canyon, through scattered western white pines, mountain hemlocks, and firs. Briefly descend the cleft of a seasonal drainage until the trail merges with a steep, rocky old road that leads you down to a junction east of the lake. The left-hand branch leads across the seasonal inlet to pleasant campsites along the stream bank. Veer to the right and follow the road past a large meadow to the east shore of White Rock Lake, **Lake** ~ ►3 where shady conifers line the shoreline and dramatic rock cliffs provide a rugged backdrop. Several decent campsites are spread around the lakeshore.

		MILESTONES
►1	0.0	Start at trailhead
►2	5.2	Summit of Mount Lola
►3	7.2	White Rock Lake

Sagehen Creek

Wildflower season reaches a dramatic crescendo in early summer along Sagehen Creek, where a short, easy trail provides access for young and old alike. Those who hike all the way to the end of the trail will have the bonus of a nice view of Stampede Reservoir.

Best Time

June is the best time to view the extensive fields of wildflowers along the creek and to see Stampede Reservoir without a bathtub ring. Mid-October is when aspens and shrubs are ablaze with fall colors.

Finding the Trail

From I-80 near the town of Truckee, travel north on CA 89 for 6.8 miles to a dirt parking area on the right, just past a highway bridge over Sagehen Creek.

Logistics

Though the trailhead is unmarked, the start of the well-worn trail is easy to locate.

Trail Description

►1 Head downstream on the north side of Sagehen Creek along the edge of a mixed forest of lodgepole pines, Jeffrey pines, white firs, incense cedars, and junipers. Lush riparian vegetation fills the creek bottom to your right, along with a wide variety of wildflowers, including lupine, aster, paintbrush, mule-ears, corn lily, senecio, penstemon, and

TRAIL USE
Hike, Run, Bike, Horses, Dogs Allowed, Child Friendly

LENGTH
5.0 miles, 2 hours

VERTICAL FEET
±225

DIFFICULTY
– **1** 2 3 4 5 +

TRAIL TYPE
Out-and-back

SURFACE TYPE
Dirt

FEATURES
Canyon
Stream
Autumn Colors
Wildflowers
Birds
Wildlife
Photo Opportunity

FACILITIES
None

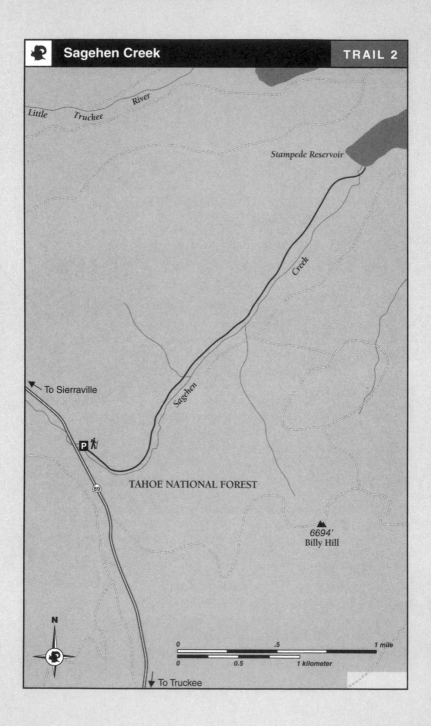

Little   Truckee   River

Stampede Reservoir

Creek

To Sierraville

Sagehen

P

TAHOE NATIONAL FOREST

89

▲
6694'
Billy Hill

N

0   .5   1 mile
0   0.5   1 kilometer

To Truckee

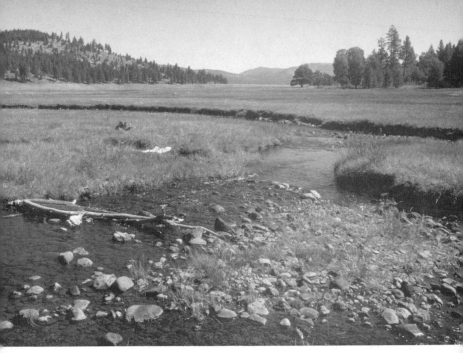

Eastern Sierra meadows *along Sagehen Creek*

buttercup. Wild rosebushes alongside the trail provide delicate pink blossoms and a sweet fragrance
in midsummer. Meadowlands farther downstream
beckon skilled botanists and curious youngsters
alike to wander off the trail and explore the lush
surroundings.

 Wildflowers

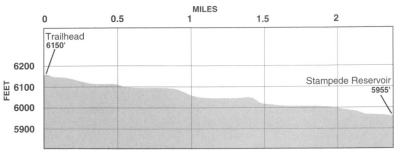

TRAIL 2 Sagehen Creek Elevation Profile

The short, easy trail along Sagehen Creek provides access to one of the finest wildflower displays in the greater Tahoe area.

Stream

Eventually, the trail veers to the northeast and moves a little farther away from the creek. You stroll through a forest of mostly lodgepole pines, where, in early summer, a bounty of mule-ears carpets the slopes with a stunning display of yellow that stretches for quite a distance. Careful observation of the hillside above reveals that this area has seen past logging and at least one forest fire. Two miles from the trailhead you traverse a grassy clearing, cross a small rivulet, and emerge into a broad meadow filled with sagebrush and grasses that borders the southeast arm of Stampede Reservoir. The trail follows a raised finger of ground above the sometimes-boggy meadow to a small copse of pines, where an old timber beam provides a way across the main channel of Sagehen Creek. The trail continues alongside the creek for a short distance before disappearing for good in the meadowland. Rimmed by pine-dotted hills, the sapphire blue waters of Stampede Reservoir stretch out in front of you. ▶2

🚶 MILESTONES

▶1	0.0	Start at trailhead
▶2	2.5	Stampede Reservoir

Summit Lake, Frog Lake Overlook, and Warren Lake

Two scenic lakes and a spectacular vista point are the principal attractions of this hike, which is within the proposed Castle Peak Wilderness. The hike to Summit Lake is an easy 2-mile stroll, whereas the trip to Warren Lake is another story—over the course of 7.5 miles you gain and lose nearly 4,500 feet of elevation. In between, Frog Lake Overlook provides a grand vista of the Donner Pass region. With three such worthwhile goals, you can tailor your trip to fit your individual needs and schedule.

Best Time

Mid-July–August is the best time for hiking on snow-free trails, though following winters of heavy snowfall, the trail across the upper basin of North Fork Prosser Creek may see lingering snowbanks well into summer.

Finding the Trail

West of Donner Summit, take the Castle Peak/Boreal Ridge Road exit from I-80. Drive to the frontage road on the south side of the freeway and proceed east 0.3 mile to the Pacific Crest Trail (PCT) parking area. The large parking lot has trailer parking, pit toilets, and running water in season.

TRAIL USE
Hike, Horses, Dogs Allowed
LENGTH*
VERTICAL FEET*
DIFFICULTY*
*See table below
TRAIL TYPE
Out-and-back
SURFACE TYPE
Dirt

FEATURES
Canyon
Mountain
Lake
Birds
Great Views
Photo Opportunity
Camping
Steep

FACILITIES
Restrooms
Picnic Tables
Water

DESTINATIONS	LENGTH	VERTICAL FEET	DIFFICULTY
SUMMIT LAKE	4.0 miles, 2 hours	±450	– 1 2 3 4 5 +
FROG LAKE OVERLOOK	8.0 miles, 5 hours	±1,700	– 1 2 3 4 5 +
WARREN LAKE	15.0 miles, 10 hours	±2,225	– 1 2 3 4 5 +

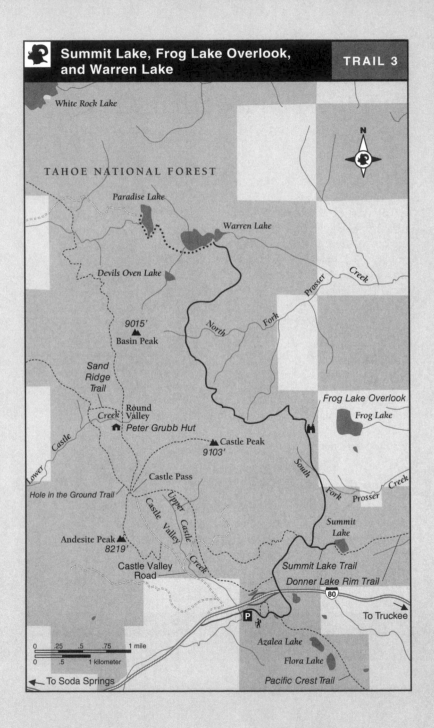

Summit Lake, Frog Lake Overlook, and Warren Lake

TRAIL 3

White Rock Lake

TAHOE NATIONAL FOREST

Paradise Lake

Warren Lake

Devils Oven Lake

Prosser Creek

North Fork

9015'
Basin Peak

Sand Ridge Trail

Frog Lake Overlook

Frog Lake

Round Valley

Castle Creek

Peter Grubb Hut

Castle Peak
9103'

Lower Castle

Castle Pass

Hole in the Ground Trail

South Fork Prosser Creek

Upper Castle Valley

Castle Valley Creek

Summit Lake

Andesite Peak
8219'

Castle Valley Road

Summit Lake Trail

Donner Lake Rim Trail

80

To Truckee

P

Azalea Lake

Flora Lake

Pacific Crest Trail

0   .25   .5   .75   1 mile
0   .5   1 kilometer

To Soda Springs

Logistics

Avoid the temptation to shorten your trip by beginning at the westbound Donner Summit Rest Area parking lot. Vehicles parked there longer than a couple of hours are subject to fines.

Trail Description

▶1 From the parking lot follow a well-signed gravel path to a stone bridge over a seasonal stream and continue on dirt track through lodgepole pines, western white pines, and white firs. Soon encounter a junction with the Glacier Meadow Loop, ▶2 where you veer right and continue eastbound toward the Pacific Crest Trail. After a short distance you come to a second junction with the Glacier Meadow Loop, ▶3 where you veer to the right again. Pass by a shallow pond, where mountain hemlocks join the mixed forest, and then make a short descent to the Pacific Crest Trail junction, near the edge of a grass- and willow-filled meadow, 0.5 mile from the trailhead. ▶4

Head north on the PCT around the fringe of the meadow and pass through a pair of large culverts underneath the eastbound and westbound lanes of I-80. Beyond the culverts you make a moderate

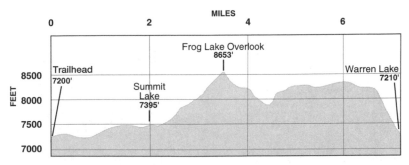

TRAIL 3   Summit Lake, Frog Lake Overlook, & Warren Lake Elevation Profile

climb to the crossing of a seasonal creek and then come to a well-signed, four-way junction, 1 mile from the trailhead. ►5

Following signed directions for Summit and Warren Lakes, turn right and proceed on a mild to moderate climb through alternating stretches of mixed forest and open areas sprinkled with granite slabs and boulders. At 1.7 miles, just past a small meadow covered with corn lilies, you come to a junction with the Donner Lake Rim Trail. ►6

To visit Summit Lake, follow the right-hand trail out of the forest and across the slopes of a granite ridge carpeted with pinemat manzanita, where views temporarily open up of the Donner Summit region. Eventually the trail heads back into the forest and leads you onward to the shoreline of serene Summit

Lake 〰️ Lake. ►7 Except for cliffs at the north end, the lake is surrounded by trees and edged with shrubs.

OPTIONS

Cross-Country Routes

Several use trails and cross-country routes in the Castle Peak backcountry provide numerous diversions. About 0.8 mile before Warren Lake, a use trail leaves the Warren Lake Trail at a low ridge, northbound for Devils Oven Lake. From there, cross-country routes proceed to Warren and Paradise Lakes. A fine loop trip returns to the trailhead by heading west from Paradise Lake on a jeep road for 1.1 miles and then following the Pacific Crest Trail (PCT) south for 8.3 miles.

Peak baggers may be tempted by a route that exits the use trail to Devils Oven Lake a short distance from the junction with the Warren Lake Trail and then ascends Basin Peak. Following a use trail along the crest of the ridge between Basin and Castle Peaks may also be rewarding. From the summit of Castle Peak, proceed along the west ridge to a connection with the PCT at Castle Pass (see Trail 5, page 48).

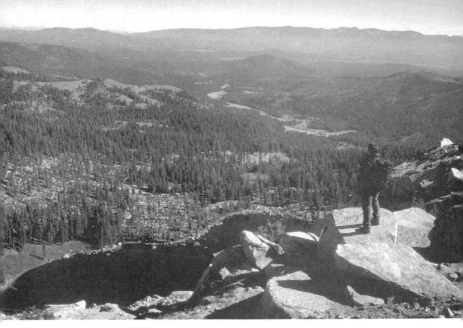

Frog Lake *from overlook*

From the Donner Lake Rim Trail junction to Summit Lake ▶8, head north on a steep climb up a forested hill toward the top of a volcanic ridge directly west of Peak 7,888. Before you reach the top, the forest gives way to shrub-covered slopes, which allows for fine views of the surrounding terrain. Beyond this point the stiff ascent temporarily abates as you stroll through a clearing and drop to a crossing of a tributary of South Fork Prosser Creek. All too soon you resume the steep climb toward a saddle just west of Peak 8,653, hopping over several more small creeks on the way. Nearing the saddle, a short use trail branches away from Warren Lake Trail and ascends rocky slopes to the top of this peak. Standing at the edge of Frog Lake Cliff, ▶9 you have a dramatic view straight down into privately owned Frog Lake, as well as west toward Castle Peak and east to the distant Carson Range.

 Steep

Indefatigable super-hikers may elect to continue their journey to Warren Lake, though a reasonable assessment of the trip will lead most recreationists to conclude that a visit to the lake is best done as a two- to three-day backpack. From the saddle, follow the trail on a winding descent across mostly open slopes dotted with conifers. At 4.4 miles reach the crest of a minor ridge and a faint junction with an old trail from the vicinity of Frog Lake. Veer west and continue the descent for 0.6 mile to the bottom of Coon Canyon. From there follow an undulating 1.5-mile traverse around the head of North Fork Prosser Creek basin to a saddle due south of Warren Lake. Beyond the saddle the trail plummets more than 1,000 feet in a mile to reach the south shore of Warren Lake. ▶10

🚶 MILESTONES

▶1	0.0	Start at Pacific Crest Trail Trailhead
▶2	0.2	Veer right at Glacier Meadow Loop junction
▶3	0.3	Veer right again at Glacier Meadow Loop junction
▶4	0.5	Turn left (north) at Pacific Crest Trail junction
▶5	1.0	Turn right (northeast) at Summit Lake Trail junction
▶6	1.7	Turn right (east) at Warren Lake Trail junction
▶7	2.0	Summit Lake
▶8	2.3	Return to Warren Lake junction, turn right (north)
▶9	4.0	Frog Lake Overlook
▶10	7.5	Warren Lake

Castle Peak

A climb to one of north Tahoe's highest summits provides summiteers with an expansive view of the northern Sierra, which on clear days includes distant Lassen Peak in the north and the coastal hills to the west.

Best Time

Mid-July–early September is the prime time for an ascent. Though this is a favorite winter ascent of backcountry skiers and snowshoers, most of the lingering snowbanks across the trail have disappeared by mid-July.

Finding the Trail

West of Donner Summit, take the Castle Peak/Boreal Ridge Road exit from I-80. Drive to the frontage road on the south side of the freeway and proceed east 0.3 mile to the Pacific Crest Trail (PCT) parking area. The large parking lot has trailer parking, pit toilets, and running water in season.

Logistics

Two alternatives will shorten the trip. The first option is to park near the start of the Castle Valley Road, just north of the I-80 ramps, and walk the road to Castle Pass. With a high-clearance vehicle, the second option is to drive the Castle Valley Road to a parking area near the Hole in the Ground Trailhead. From there a shorter hike along the road leads to Castle Pass.

TRAIL USE
Hike, Dogs Allowed

LENGTH
9.6 miles, 3 hours

VERTICAL FEET
±2,205

DIFFICULTY
– 1 2 3 4 **5** +

TRAIL TYPE
Out-and-back

SURFACE TYPE
Dirt

FEATURES
Canyon
Mountain
Summit
Wildflowers
Great Views
Photo Opportunity

FACILITIES
Restrooms
Picnic Tables
Water

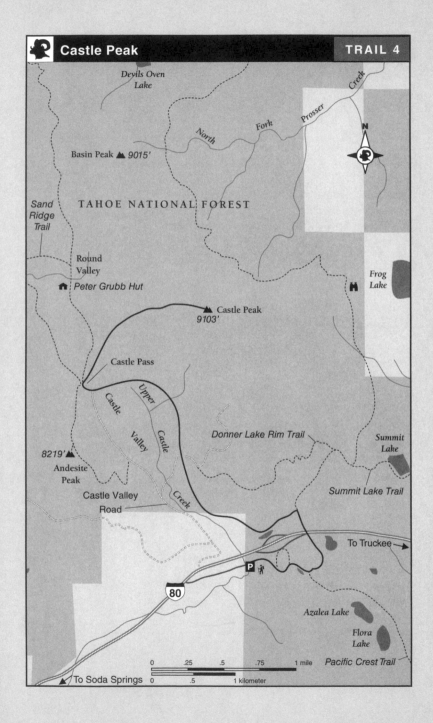

Devils Oven
Lake

Prosser   Creek

North   Fork

N

Basin Peak ▲ 9015'

*Sand
Ridge
Trail*

TAHOE NATIONAL FOREST

Round
Valley

Frog
Lake

⌂ Peter Grubb Hut

▲ Castle Peak
9103'

Castle Pass

Upper

Castle

Castle Valley

Donner Lake Rim Trail

*Summit
Lake*

8219' ▲

Andesite
Peak

Summit Lake Trail

Castle Valley
Road

Creek

To Truckee →

P 🚶

80

Azalea Lake

*Flora
Lake*

Pacific Crest Trail

| 0 | .25 | .5 | .75 | 1 mile |
| 0 | | .5 | | 1 kilometer |

▲ To Soda Springs

Trail Description

▶1 From the parking lot follow a well-signed gravel path to a stone bridge over a seasonal stream and continue on dirt track through lodgepole pines, western white pines, and white firs. Soon encounter a junction with the Glacier Meadow Loop, ▶2 where you veer right and continue eastbound toward the Pacific Crest Trail. After a short distance you come to a second junction with the Glacier Meadow Loop, ▶3 where you veer to the right again. Pass by a shallow pond, where mountain hemlocks join the mixed forest, and then make a short descent to the Pacific Crest Trail junction, near the edge of a grass- and willow-filled meadow, 0.5 mile from the trailhead. ▶4

Head north on the PCT around the fringe of the meadow and pass through a pair of large culverts, underneath the eastbound and westbound lanes of I-80. Beyond the culverts you make a moderate climb to the crossing of a seasonal creek and then come to a well-signed, four-way junction, 1 mile from the trailhead. ▶5

Remaining on the Pacific Crest Trail, you proceed straight ahead at the four-way junction, following signed directions to Castle Pass. The PCT rises and then drops to the north shore of a small pond, where you should veer right at an unmarked

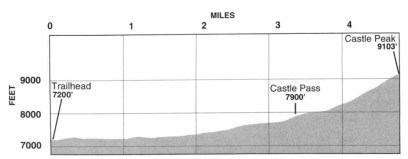

TRAIL 4 Castle Peak Elevation Profile

Cross-Country Routes

OPTIONS

Ambitious peak baggers can double summit by following a boot-beaten path from Castle Peak along the north ridge to the top of 9,017-foot Basin Peak. On the way back, dropping west from the ridge about halfway between Castle and Basin Peaks to head cross-country to a connection with the Pacific Crest Trail in Round Valley provides an easier alternative to a return over Castle Peak.

Y-junction with a path bound for the Donner Summit Rest Area.

Beyond the unmarked junction, you follow mildly graded trail through mixed forest, toward Castle Valley. Eventually the trail brings you alongside the creek for a brief time and then travels just east of the verdant meadows of Castle Valley. Use trails branch away from the PCT at various points, headed toward the creek and meadows. At 2.3 miles from the trailhead you cross a well-traveled dirt road, and then continue upstream through Castle Valley, hopping over lushly lined tributaries along the way. Nearing the head of the valley, the PCT bends to the west on an ascending traverse to a signed three-way junction with a trail from the Castle Valley Road. ▶6 From there, a short but stiff climb brings you to Castle Pass and a junction with a trio of paths, 3.3 miles from the trailhead. ▶7

At Castle Pass take the use trail to the right, which ascends the west ridge of Castle Peak. As you climb the rocky ridge the conifers diminish, allowing you increasingly good views of Castle Peak ahead and other peaks and landmarks scattered around the Donner Pass region. A steep, zigzagging ascent heads around to the north side of the mountain, where switchbacks then lead you toward the summit. After a rocky stretch of climbing, a splendid view greets you at the top of the

 Summit

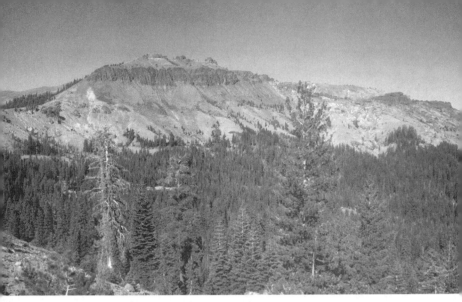

Castle Peak

9,103-foot peak. ▶8 Clear days offer a 360-degree view, all the way to Lassen Peak in the north, Mount Diablo and the coastal hills to the west, the peaks of Desolation Wilderness to the south, and the Carson Range to the east. Don't forget to pack along a map of the area to help you identify the numerous landmarks visible from the summit.

🚶 MILESTONES

▶1	0.0	Start at Pacific Crest Trail Trailhead
▶2	0.2	Veer right at Glacier Meadow Loop junction
▶3	0.3	Veer right again at Glacier Meadow Loop junction
▶4	0.5	Turn left (north) at PCT junction
▶5	1.0	Proceed straight ahead (west) at Summit Lake Trail junction
▶6	3.2	Veer right at Castle Valley Road junction
▶7	3.3	Castle Pass, leave PCT and turn right on use trail
▶8	4.8	Summit of Castle Peak

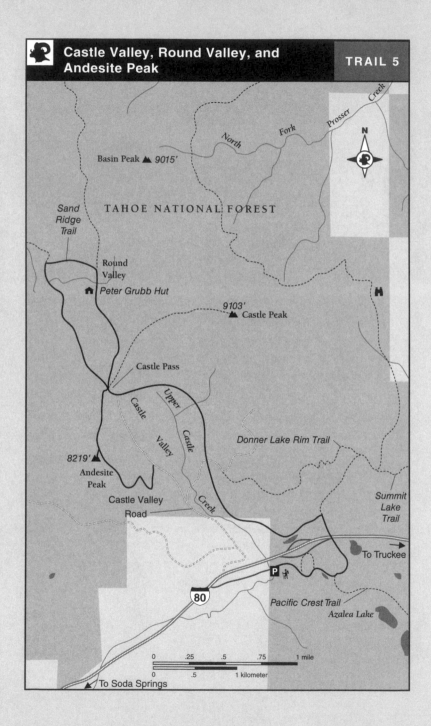

Basin Peak ▲ 9015'

North Fork

Prosser Creek

N

TAHOE NATIONAL FOREST

Sand Ridge Trail

Round Valley

⌂ Peter Grubb Hut

9103'
▲ Castle Peak

Castle Pass

Upper
Castle
Castle
Valley

Donner Lake Rim Trail

8219' ▲
Andesite Peak

Castle Valley Road

Creek

Summit Lake Trail

To Truckee

P ⚥

Pacific Crest Trail

Azalea Lake

80

0   .25   .5   .75   1 mile

0   .5   1 kilometer

▲ To Soda Springs

Castle Valley, Round Valley, and Andesite Peak

Though most of this route travels outside the proposed Castle Peak Wilderness, plenty of pleasant terrain is encountered along the way, including two picturesque meadows and an excellent view from atop Andesite Peak. Both Castle and Round meadows offer the chance to see raptors in search of prey or deer browsing the tender foliage. Throw in the Peter Grubb Hut for a bit of Tahoe Sierra history and you have the makings of a fine adventure.

Best Time

Mid-July–September generally provides snow-free hiking.

Finding the Trail

West of Donner Summit, take the Castle Peak/Boreal Ridge Road exit from I-80. Drive to the frontage road on the south side of the freeway and proceed east 0.3 mile to the Pacific Crest Trail (PCT) parking area. The large parking lot has trailer parking, pit toilets, and running water in season.

Logistics

With a pair of durable vehicles you can arrange a shuttle and shave off 1.6 miles of hiking by driving the Castle Valley Road to within 0.1 mile of the Hole in the Ground Trailhead. With a high-clearance vehicle you may be able to get all the way to the trailhead.

The trip length with a shuttle is 8.0 miles.

TRAIL USE
Hike, Run, Bike,
Horses, Dogs Allowed,
Child Friendly
LENGTH
9.6 miles, 6.5 hours
VERTICAL FEET
±1,700
DIFFICULTY
– 1 2 **3** 4 5 +
TRAIL TYPE
Loop
SURFACE TYPE
Dirt

FEATURES
Canyon
Mountain
Summit
Wildflowers
Wildlife
Great Views
Historical Interest
Camping
Steep

FACILITIES
Restrooms
Picnic Tables
Water

Trail Description

►1 From the parking lot follow a well-signed gravel path to a stone bridge over a seasonal stream and continue on dirt track through lodgepole pines, western white pines, and white firs. Soon encounter a junction with the Glacier Meadow Loop, ►2 where you veer right and continue eastbound toward the Pacific Crest Trail. After a short distance you come to a second junction with the Glacier Meadow Loop, ►3 where you veer to the right again. Pass by a shallow pond, where mountain hemlocks join the mixed forest, and then make a short descent to the Pacific Crest Trail junction, near the edge of a grass- and willow-filled meadow, 0.5 mile from the trailhead. ►4

Head north on the PCT around the fringe of the meadow and pass through a pair of large culverts, underneath the eastbound and westbound lanes of I-80. Beyond the culverts you make a moderate climb to the crossing of a seasonal creek and then come to a well-signed, four-way junction, 1 mile from the trailhead. ►5

Remaining on the Pacific Crest Trail, you proceed straight ahead at the four-way junction, following signed directions to Castle Pass. The PCT rises and

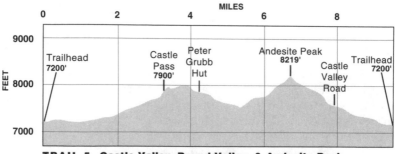

TRAIL 5 Castle Valley, Round Valley, & Andesite Peak Elevation Profile

then drops to the north shore of a small pond, where you should veer right at an unmarked Y-junction with a path bound for the Donner Summit Rest Area.

Beyond the unmarked junction, you follow mildly graded trail through mixed forest, toward Castle Valley. Eventually the trail brings you along-side the creek for a brief time and then travels just east of the verdant meadows of Castle Valley. Use trails branch away from the PCT at various points, headed toward the creek and meadows. At 2.3 miles from the trailhead you cross a well-traveled dirt road, and then continue upstream through Castle Valley, hopping over a number of lushly lined tribu-taries along the way. Nearing the head of the valley, the PCT bends to the west on an ascending traverse to a signed three-way junction with a trail from the Castle Valley Road. ▶6 From there, a short but stiff climb brings you to Castle Pass and a five-way junc-tion, 3.3 miles from the trailhead. ▶7

 Steep

At Castle Pass, proceed north on the Pacific Crest Trail, on a traverse across a lightly forested slope. After about 0.5 mile you begin a moder-ate, switchbacking descent toward Round Valley.

OPTION

Peter Grubb Hut

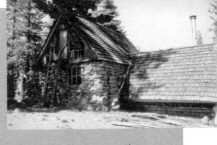

The Peter Grubb Hut, built in the 1930s, was the northernmost in a series of six huts planned for the Tahoe Sierra along the crest between Donner and Echo Passes. The huts were patterned after hut systems in the Swiss Alps. The four huts that were built have provided overnight shelter at a nominal cost for backcountry skiers and hikers for several decades. For more information or to make a reservation, contact the Sierra Club at 530-426-3632.

**Historical
Interest**
Nearing the floor of the valley, a short use trail
leads to the Peter Grubb Hut, ►8 4.2 miles from the
PCT Trailhead. The hut is complete with a wood-
burning stove, firewood, gas stove, cooking utensils,
table and chairs, a loft with sleeping platforms, and
a detached outhouse. Interesting old photos and
memorabilia cover the walls and provide a sample
of the area's history.

The PCT crosses Lower Castle Creek north of the
hut and leads to a Y-junction with the Sand Ridge
Trail a short way farther, where you leave the PCT
and turn left (east). ►9 A winding descent through
a mixed forest of western white pines, red firs, and
lodgepole pines follows, leading across some lushly
lined streams and below a striking granite cliff to
another Y-junction with the Hole in the Ground
Trail, 0.6 mile from the previous junction. ►10

Turn left (south) at the junction, on a moderately graded, winding descent through mixed forest, to a small, willow-filled meadow bordered with
wildflowers, and proceed to a crossing of Lower
Castle Creek. Beyond the crossing you make a
moderately steep, winding climb toward the crest of
a hill and then follow gently rising trail toward the
vicinity of Castle Pass, where you reach a junction
with a short connecting trail to the PCT, 6 miles
from the trailhead. ►11

Great Views
Continue to climb toward the north ridge of
Andesite Peak. Where you gain the crest of the ridge,
Castle Peak and Valley burst into view. Follow the
crest toward Andesite Peak, reaching a Y-junction
with the 0.1-mile spur trail to the summit, at 6.5
miles in. ►12 The short climb to the top of Andesite
Peak is rewarded by a fine 360-degree view. ►13

From the summit of Andesite Peak, return to
the junction. ►14 Follow the Hole in the Ground
Trail on a switchbacking descent across a forested
hillside toward Castle Valley below. The forest parts
temporarily to allow one more view of Castle Peak

and the Carson Range to the east. You're soon back into the forest, where a series of switchbacks leads you down the hillside to the floor of the valley and a junction with the Castle Valley Road at 7.9 miles. ▶15 Near a couple of trailhead signs, a small patch of dirt provides parking for any high-clearance vehicles that make it this far up the road.

Without a vehicle at the trailhead you should head southeast and follow a rough and rocky section of the road for about 0.1 mile to a second parking area suitable for sedans. Without a vehicle parked here you must continue down the valley all the way to the end of the Castle Valley Road, walk the paved access road below I-80 to the frontage road on the south side, and follow that road back to the trailhead. ▶16

🚶	**MILESTONES**	
▶1	0.0	Start at Pacific Crest Trail Trailhead
▶2	0.2	Veer right at Glacier Meadow Loop junction
▶3	0.3	Veer right again at Glacier Meadow Loop junction
▶4	0.5	Turn left (north) at PCT junction
▶5	1.0	Proceed straight ahead (west) at Summit Lake Trail junction
▶6	3.2	Veer right at Castle Valley Road junction
▶7	3.3	Castle Pass, proceed north on PCT
▶8	4.2	Peter Grubb Hut
▶9	4.4	Turn left (west) at junction with Sand Ridge Trail
▶10	5.0	Turn left (south) at junction with Hole in the Ground Trail
▶11	6.0	Proceed straight ahead (south) at junction with Castle Pass lateral
▶12	6.5	Junction with trail to Andesite Peak
▶13	6.6	Andesite Peak
▶14	6.7	Junction with trail to Andesite Peak
▶15	7.9	Turn right (southeast) onto Castle Valley Road
▶16	9.6	Return to PCT Trailhead

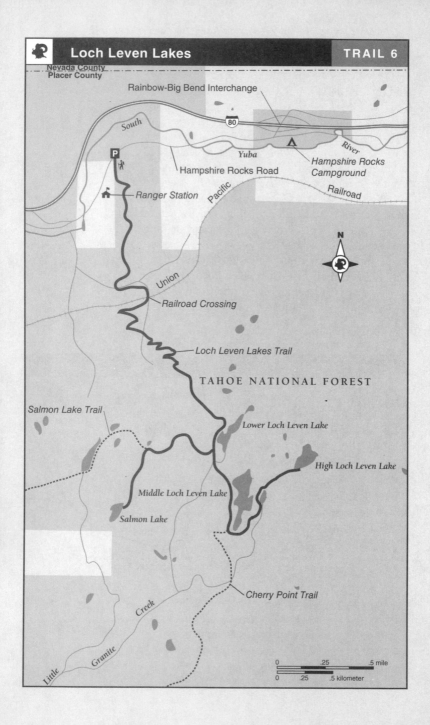

Nevada County
Placer County

Rainbow-Big Bend Interchange

80

South

Yuba

Hampshire Rocks Road

Ranger Station

Pacific

Hampshire Rocks Campground

Railroad

N

Union

Railroad Crossing

Loch Leven Lakes Trail

TAHOE NATIONAL FOREST

Salmon Lake Trail

Lower Loch Leven Lake

High Loch Leven Lake

Middle Loch Leven Lake

Salmon Lake

Cherry Point Trail

Creek

Little

Granite

0   .25   .5 mile
0   .25   .5 kilometer

Loch Leven Lakes

The Loch Leven Lakes provide hikers itching for summer an early-season opportunity to reach a trio of picturesque lakes nestled into a granite basin. A pleasant side trip to Salmon Lake increases the number of lakes to four. Swimmers will appreciate the relatively warm waters and scads of slabs and islands for sunbathing, while anglers can test their skills on the stocked trout that inhabit the lakes.

Best Time

A low-elevation trail by Tahoe Sierra standards, the Loch Leven Lakes Trail is usually snow-free by mid- to late June, when wildflowers along the lower section of trail are at their glorious peak. Cool but pleasant weather usually persists into November.

Finding the Trail

Take the Rainbow Road/Big Bend exit from I-80 and follow Hampshire Rocks Road westbound for 0.9 mile to the trailhead parking area on the right-hand shoulder. The trail begins on the opposite side of the road from the parking lot.

Logistics

The alignment of the Loch Leven Lakes Trail is incorrectly shown on the USGS *Cisco Grove* quadrangle. The map on the facing page shows the true route.

TRAIL USE
Hike, Run, Bike,
Horses, Dogs Allowed

LENGTH
8.0 miles, 4 hours

VERTICAL FEET
±1,710

DIFFICULTY
– 1 2 3 **4** 5 +

TRAIL TYPE
Out-and-back

SURFACE TYPE
Dirt

FEATURES
Canyon
Mountain
Lake
Wildflowers
Photo Opportunity
Camping

FACILITIES
Restrooms

Trail Description

▶1 An old wood sign marked LOCH LEVEN LAKES is all that delineates the start of a trail that climbs over a shrub- and boulder-covered hillside of exposed granite slabs beneath widely scattered conifers. A short, winding descent takes you briefly into a stand of white firs and lodgepole pines with a lush understory before the climbing resumes across mostly open terrain with nice views of Cisco Butte and the South Yuba River Canyon. Soon the trail leads back into a grove of trees with a small pond that turns into little more than a quagmire by late summer. Beyond the pond, cross another stretch of shrubs and granite slabs before dropping through another forested section to a bridge across an alder-lined stream. Beyond the bridge a steep 0.25-mile climb leads to the twin tracks of the Union Pacific Railroad, 1.25 miles from the trailhead. ▶2 As you cross the two sets of tracks pay close attention to traffic, especially coming toward you from the uphill direction, as trains descending from Donner Pass move swiftly and relatively quietly.

Find the continuation of the trail on the far side of the tracks and resume climbing through a mixed forest of incense cedars; white firs; and Jeffrey, lodgepole, and western white pines. Soon you reach the first of many switchbacks that will eventually transport you out of the South Yuba River Canyon

Canyon

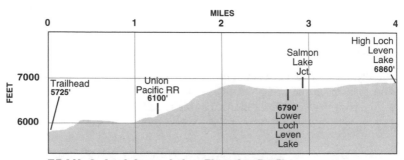

TRAIL 6 Loch Leven Lakes Elevation Profile

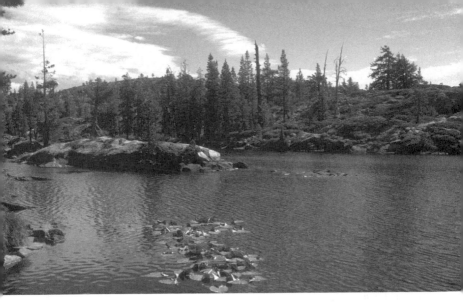

Lower *Loch Leven Lake*

and into the lakes basin. Approaching Loch Leven Summit, the high point of the climb, the gradient mercifully eases and you follow a slight descent into the lakes basin until a short, steep, and rocky section of trail brings you to the first of the lakes. An old sign heralds your arrival at the west shore of Loch Leven Lake, 2.75 miles from the trailhead. ▶3 Passable campsites are scattered around the lake and gently sloping granite slabs are sure to lure swimmers and sunbathers. Continue along the west side of Lower Loch Leven Lake to an unsigned junction with a lateral to Salmon Lake (see page 58).

 Lake

OPTION

Rainbow Lodge

Halfway between the trailhead and the freeway, Rainbow Lodge provides an excellent watering hole or eatery after a trip to Loch Leven Lakes. Fine bed-and-breakfast packages are available for those looking for an overnight adventure. Call 800-500-3871 or visit the website at **royalgorge.com** for more information.

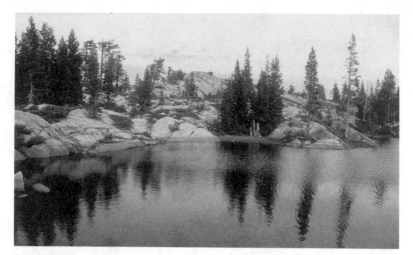

Salmon Lake

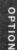

Side Trip to Salmon Lake

From Lower Loch Leven Lake, follow the unsigned side trail right on a rising and winding climb across grass- and flower-covered slopes for 0.3 mile, followed by a gradual descent through alternating sections of granite slabs and light forest. Just before the lake, you reach a junction with a trail heading west to the Salmon Lake Trailhead on Huysink Lake Road. ►4 Veer left at the junction and continue another 0.2 mile to Salmon Lake. Though smaller and not as scenic as the Loch Leven Lakes, Salmon Lake is rimmed by low granite humps, scattered trees, and clumps of shrubs and grasses. Backpackers will find more solitude than at Loch Leven but far fewer campsites. This side trip adds 1.8 miles to the main route.

Camping

From the Salmon Lake junction, ►4 a brief descent followed by a short climb leads to Middle Loch Leven Lake, where a number of pleasant campsites will lure overnighters. At the far end of the lake is a junction with the Cherry Point Trail, which heads southwest toward North Fork American River. ►5

Turn left at the junction and follow the trail around the lower end of the middle lake, ascend a rock cleft, and then climb over granite slabs to the upper lake. ▶6 High Loch Leven Lake is perhaps the most picturesque of the lakes, with heather-rimmed shores bordered by granite cliffs and stands of conifers. Fine campsites above the southeast shore will certainly appeal to those backpackers willing to hike all the way to the last lake in the chain.

 Photo Opportunity

🚶	**MILESTONES**	
▶1	0.0	Start at trailhead
▶2	1.25	Union Pacific Railroad tracks
▶3	2.75	Lower Loch Leven Lake
▶4	2.9	Proceed straight ahead (south) at Salmon Lake junction
▶5	3.3	Veer left (east) at Cherry Point Trail junction
▶6	4.0	High Loch Leven Lake

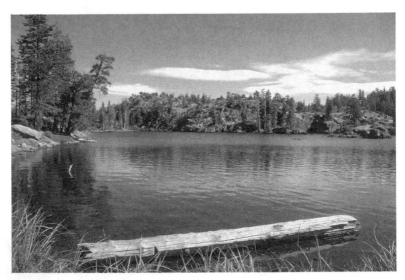

Middle *Loch Leven Lake*

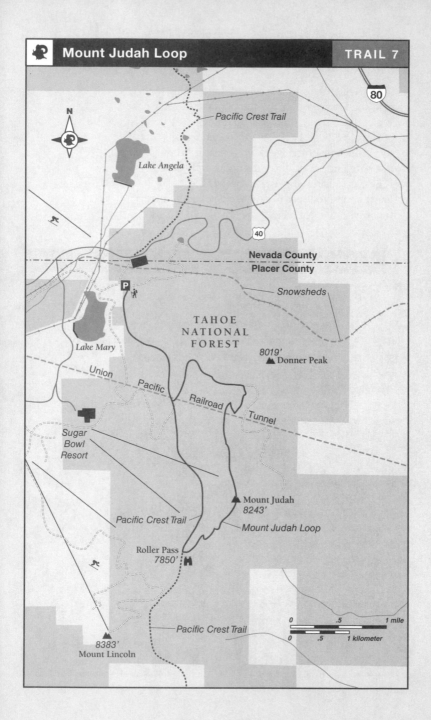

Mount Judah Loop

TRAIL 7

80

Pacific Crest Trail

N

Lake Angela

40

Nevada County
Placer County

P

Snowsheds

TAHOE
NATIONAL
FOREST

Lake Mary

8019'
▲ Donner Peak

Union Pacific Railroad

Tunnel

Sugar
Bowl
Resort

▲ Mount Judah
8243'

Pacific Crest Trail

Mount Judah Loop

Roller Pass
7850'

Pacific Crest Trail

0   .5   1 mile
0   .5   1 kilometer

8383'
Mount Lincoln

Mount Judah Loop

With minimal effort, hikers can reach some of the grandest views available in the northern Tahoe Sierra, via the 4.6-mile Mount Judah Loop. The rugged terrain around Donner Pass is impressive, and the trail affords many excellent vista points along the way to the awe-inspiring view from the summit of Mount Judah. The section of the loop that connects with the Pacific Crest Trail (PCT) was constructed in the 1990s, but despite its recent origin, the Mount Judah Loop has justifiably become a very popular hike, so don't anticipate a high degree of solitude. Be sure to pack plenty of water, as none is available en route.

Best Time

The trail is generally snow-free mid-July–October, though early in the season lingering snowbanks may cover the forested sections of trail, particularly following winters of heavy snows.

Finding the Trail

From I-80 take either the Donner Lake or Soda Springs exit and drive approximately 4 miles on Donner Pass Road (Old Highway 40) to Donner Pass. Near the pass, turn south onto an old road, observing PACIFIC CREST TRAIL signs. After a short distance, turn left and immediately reach the trailhead, where you'll find very limited parking.

TRAIL USE
Hike, Run, Horses,
Dogs Allowed,
Child Friendly

LENGTH
4.6 miles, 2.5 hours

VERTICAL FEET
±1,165

DIFFICULTY
– 1 2 **3** 4 5 +

TRAIL TYPE
Loop

SURFACE TYPE
Dirt

FEATURES
Mountain
Summit
Great Views

FACILITIES
None

Logistics

Though the Mount Judah Loop is outside of a designated wilderness, mountain bikes are not allowed on the Pacific Crest Trail.

Trail Description

▶1 After a narrow swath of lush vegetation filled with flowers and ferns, a series of short switchbacks leads you on a climb of a pine- and fir-dotted granite headwall. Beyond the switchbacks, follow the trail across a hillside carpeted with huckleberry oak, where views of the Donner Pass region improve with each step (the lake directly below you is Lake Mary). After a while, pass through a stand of red firs before breaking back out into the open at a crossing of a ski slope. In this clearing, 0.9 mile from the trailhead, you encounter a junction between the PCT and the north end of the Mount Judah Loop. ▶2

Remaining on the PCT, you pass below a chairlift for the Sugar Bowl Ski Area, and then cross an old road, 0.1 mile from the junction. Reenter forest beyond the road, where mountain hemlocks begin to intermix with the red firs, and, in early summer, mule-ears provide bursts of color. Reach the south

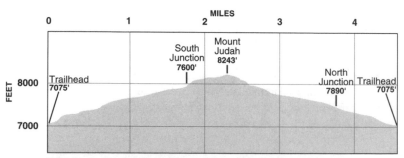

TRAIL 7 Mount Judah Loop Elevation Profile

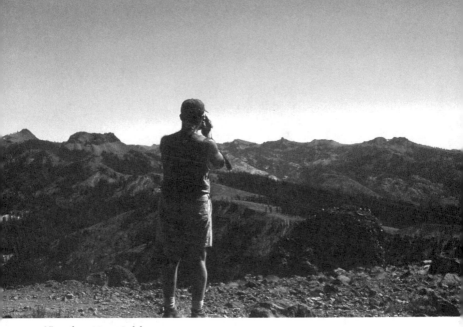

View *from Mount Judah*

junction of the Mount Judah Loop at 1.8 miles from the trailhead. ▶3

Leave the PCT and follow the loop trail on a winding ascent of Mount Judah's southwest ridge, reaching the top of the peak at 0.5 mile from the junction. At the time of research, a large cairn with metal flagpole and tattered flags marked the summit. ▶4 The marvelous view includes such landmarks as Donner Lake, Martis Valley, and the Carson Range to the east; Castle Peak, Mount Lola, and the Sierra Buttes to the north; Sugar Bowl, Summit Valley, and Lake Van Norden to the west; and the continuation of the Sierra Crest to the south.

 Great Views

From the top of Mount Judah, descend a bare ridge to a saddle and then start climbing again toward the north summit. The trail veers east away from this slightly lower peak, though a short use trail branching away from the main trail provides an easy way to the top. Traverse the east side of the ridge before a descent leads through a mixed forest around the nose of the ridge to a three-way junction at a saddle between Mount Judah and Donner Peak, 3.1 miles from the trailhead. ►5

Summit ◬

With extra time and energy you could follow a use trail from the saddle, northeast to the base of Donner Peak's multiple summit pinnacles. However, from there you'll need some basic rock climbing skills to scramble up exfoliating slabs to the top of the easiest summit.

From the junction, bend left and follow the course of an old road for 0.4 mile on a steady descent around the north side of the mountain to the resumption of singletrack trail. Heading southwest, you continue the descent into a thickening forest until reaching the ski slope and the north junction of the PCT, 3.7 miles from the trailhead. ►6 From there, retrace your steps 0.9 mile along the PCT to the trailhead. ►7

🚶	MILESTONES		
►1	0.0	Start at trailhead	
►2	0.9	Proceed straight ahead (south) at north loop junction	
►3	1.8	Turn left (northeast) at south loop junction	
►4	2.3	Summit of Mount Judah	
►5	3.1	Veer left (west) at three-way junction	
►6	3.7	Turn right (north) at north loop junction	
►7	4.6	Return to trailhead	

Pacific Crest Trail: Donner Pass to Squaw Valley

This section of the Pacific Crest Trail (PCT) lives up to its name, offering some of the finest views in the Tahoe area from a several-mile stretch of trail that stays on or near the actual crest of the range. The 15-mile distance may be daunting to casual hikers, but experienced hikers in good condition will find the well-maintained PCT a rewarding challenge.

Best Time

The views from the trail are impressive anytime between mid-July and October. Early in the season snowbanks may cover some of the forested sections of the trail, particularly following winters of heavy snowfalls.

Finding the Trail

START: From I-80 take either the Donner Lake or Soda Springs exit and drive approximately 4 miles on Donner Pass Road (Old Highway 40) to Donner Pass. Near the pass, just west of Alpine Skills International, turn south onto an old road, observing PACIFIC CREST TRAIL signs. After a short distance, turn left and immediately reach the trailhead, where you'll find very limited parking.

END: From CA 89, about 8.5 miles south of Truckee and 5 miles north of Tahoe City, head west on Squaw Valley Road for 2.25 miles and park in the large parking area on the right, across from the fire station and the Olympic Village Inn.

TRAIL USE
Hike, Horses

LENGTH
15.0 miles, 8–10 hours

VERTICAL FEET
+3,000/-3,800

DIFFICULTY
– 1 2 3 4 **5** +

TRAIL TYPE
Point-to-point

SURFACE TYPE
Dirt

FEATURES
Mountain
Summit
Great Views
Photo Opportunity
Camping
Secluded

FACILITIES
None

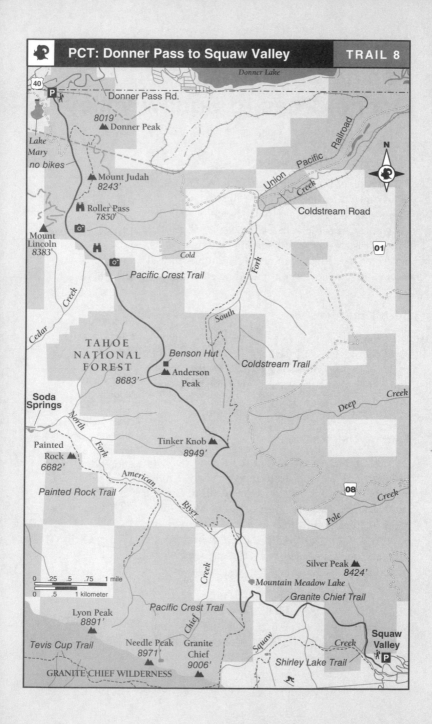

40

Donner Lake

Donner Pass Rd.

8019'
▲ Donner Peak

Lake
Mary
no bikes

▲ Mount Judah
8243'

Union   Pacific   Railroad

Creek

Coldstream Road

Roller Pass
7850'

01

Mount
Lincoln
8383'

Cold

Fork

Pacific Crest Trail

South

Cedar

Creek

TAHOE
NATIONAL
FOREST

Benson Hut

Coldstream Trail

▲ Anderson
Peak
8683'

Soda
Springs

North

Creek

Deep

Painted
Rock ▲
6682'

Fork

Tinker Knob ▲
8949'

American

08

Painted Rock Trail

River

Pole   Creek

Creek

0 .25 .5 .75 1 mile
0   .5   1 kilometer

Silver Peak ▲
8424'

● Mountain Meadow Lake

Pacific Crest Trail

Granite Chief Trail

Lyon Peak
8891'
▲

Chief

Squaw

Creek

Squaw
Valley
P

Tevis Cup Trail

Needle Peak
8971'
▲

Granite
Chief
9006'
▲

Shirley Lake Trail

GRANITE CHIEF WILDERNESS

N

Trail Description

►1 After a narrow swath of lush vegetation filled with flowers and ferns, a series of short switchbacks leads you on a climb of a pine- and fir-dotted granite headwall. Beyond the switchbacks, follow the trail across a hillside carpeted with huckleberry oak, where views of the Donner Pass region improve with each step (the lake directly below you is Lake Mary). After a while, pass through a stand of red firs before breaking back out into the open at a crossing of a ski slope. In this clearing, 0.9 mile from the trailhead, you encounter a junction between the PCT and the north end of the Mount Judah Loop. ►2

Remaining on the PCT, you pass below a chair-lift for the Sugar Bowl Ski Area, and then cross an old road, 0.1 mile from the junction. Reenter forest beyond the road, where mountain hemlocks begin to intermix with the red firs, and, in early summer, mule-ears provide bursts of color. Reach the south junction of the Mount Judah Loop at 1.8 miles from the trailhead. ►3

Remaining on the Pacific Crest Trail, continue south from the junction for a short distance to a hemlock-shaded saddle known as Roller Pass, where a metal post bears a historical marker complete with a plaque and a quotation from Nicholas Carriger,

Mountain bikes are not allowed on this section of the Pacific Crest Trail.

 Great Views

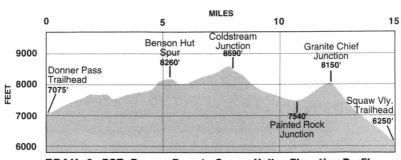

TRAIL 8 PCT: Donner Pass to Squaw Valley Elevation Profile

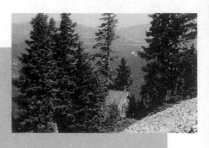

Benson Hut

Backpackers will find a dearth of
campsites along this route—the
only reasonable sites are the pair
of basins just north of the crossing of the North Fork American
River. However, overnighters may be able to obtain spartan
lodging in the Benson Hut by contacting the Sierra Club at
530-426-3632 or checking out the website at **vault.sierraclub
.org/outings/lodges/huts.**

who traveled with the ill-fated Donner Party to Salt
Lake City. In September 1846 the pioneers winched
their wagons up to this spot with the aid of oxen. A
short spur trail leads east from the saddle to the lip
above the steep wall of Emigrant Canyon and to a
vista that will certainly increase your admiration for
these rugged pioneers and their dogged determina-
tion in getting their wagons out of the deep canyon
and up to the pass.

Away from Roller Pass, the PCT closely follows
the Sierra Crest through light forest. Soon the trees
diminish, and a nearly continuous stream of awesome views begins as you traverse the east slope of
Mount Lincoln. In the middle of nowhere, an old
wood sign marked MT. LINCOLN points toward
the summit, but all evidence of a former trail has
vanished. If your desire is to scale this peak, an
easier way to the summit can be found farther south,
where a use trail leaves the PCT to follow the southeast ridge to the top.

Summit ▲

As you continue, the Sierra Crest seems to
stretch out ahead forever, while to the west the gash
created by the North Fork American River seems
too deep to be real. For the next several miles this
section of the PCT is a prototypical crest trail, as
the path stays high, either directly on or very near

the apex of the range. Heading away from Mount Lincoln, the PCT descends across an open volcanic slope, which during midsummer is covered in a sea of yellow from multitudinous mule-ears. A pair of long-legged switchbacks takes you through a stand of western white pines, red firs, and mountain hemlocks before you emerge back out into the open across shrub-covered slopes. You reach the bottom of the 0.75-mile descent from Mount Lincoln at a 7,500-foot saddle overlooking Coldstream Valley to the east and Cedar Creek Canyon to the west.

From the saddle you ascend lunarlike slopes, where only small tufts of vegetation and a few mule-ears seem capable of taking root in the porous volcanic soils. Eventually tobacco brush, currant, and sagebrush regain a foothold, as you progress toward the next high point, Anderson Peak, which from the trail presents a dramatic foreground profile. Cross a hillside covered with muddy-looking lava flows, follow a pair of switchbacks, and then pass below Peak 8,374 on the way to the base of Anderson Peak, where you'll encounter a use trail branching away from the PCT, 5.3 miles from the trailhead. ▶4

Following this unsigned path away from the PCT will take you up the north ridge of Anderson Peak in 10 minutes or so to Benson Hut, one of four historical huts operated by the Sierra Club. Unless you're caught in a life-threatening storm, advance reservations are required for use of the hut (see the sidebar on the opposite page). Peak baggers can continue on a use trail beyond the hut, which leads across a talus slope and then climbs steeply to the summit of Anderson Peak, where they'll enjoy another superb vista.

Away from the spur-trail junction to Benson Hut, the PCT skirts the west side of Anderson Peak well below the summit and follows a mile-long, gently ascending course southeast toward Tinker Knob. As you hike, tiny, drought-tolerant wildflowers

If you wish to reach the summit of Tinker Knob, leave the trail where the PCT veers sharply east, and make the easy scramble over fractured rock to the top of the 8,949-foot peak.

 Camping

cheer you onward. Just below Tinker Knob, where the PCT veers sharply east, you reach the high point of the route between Donner Pass and Squaw Valley.

Begin your 2-mile descent from Tinker Knob to the North Fork American River by turning east on a descending trail below the north face of Tinker Knob. After 0.25 mile reach the junction with the Coldstream Trail near Tinker Knob Saddle, 8.2 miles from the trailhead. ▶5 The 6-mile Coldstream Trail offers an alternate route to a remote trailhead in Coldstream Valley.

From Tinker Knob Saddle, you drop steeply via switchbacks into the canyon of a tributary to the North Fork American River. After 0.6 mile the grade eases, as you follow a descending traverse well below the crest, hopping over a pair of spring-fed streams along the way. Enter a basin where waterless campsites are available and continue to a smaller basin with both water and at least one campsite, 0.3 mile farther. Beyond the second basin a steeper descent takes you past rock outcrops to a crossing of the North Fork American River and a junction with Painted Rock Trail at 10.7 miles from the trailhead. ▶6

From the Painted Rock junction, a series of switchbacks leads you up to the crest of a ridge to good views of Granite Chief to the south and Needle and Lyon Peaks to the southwest. The USGS *Granite Chief* quad shows the old alignment of the trail that used to follow the headwaters of the North Fork

Great Views

upstream to Mountain Meadow Lake. The PCT was subsequently rerouted, as the land around the lake is privately owned and also is used by the University of California as an ecological study area. Follow this newer section of trail to a junction, about 0.4 mile directly southwest of the lake and 12.2 miles from the trailhead, where the Granite Chief Trail heads northeast. ▶7

Leave the PCT at the junction and head northeast on the Granite Chief Trail, following a winding descent through a thick forest of mountain hemlocks and red firs. Switchbacks lead into a tributary canyon of Squaw Creek, where patches of flower-filled meadow periodically interrupt the forest. Break out into the open, as you leave the trees and descend a series of sloping, granite benches that afford fine views of the Squaw Valley area. Locating the route of the trail over these granite benches may be difficult at times, but ducks and old paint blazes on rocks may help guide you.

 Wildflowers

About 1.5 miles from the PCT junction, you make an easy crossing of a perennial stream and continue the descent, through alternating stretches of light forest and granite slabs. Cross a marshy hillside fed by seeps and then follow switchbacks to the easy crossing of another Squaw Creek tributary, which you then follow downstream through thickening vegetation. Nearing the valley floor, a number of intersecting paths combined with a lack of signs create a mildly confusing conclusion to your journey, but fortunately all paths lead to the large parking lot at Squaw Valley. ►8

大	MILESTONES	
►1	0.0	Start at trailhead
►2	0.9	Proceed straight ahead (south) at north loop junction
►3	1.8	Proceed straight ahead (south) at south loop junction
►4	5.3	Spur trail to Benson Hut
►5	8.2	Proceed straight ahead (south) at Coldstream Trail junction
►6	10.7	Proceed straight ahead (south) at Painted Rock Trail junction
►7	12.2	Turn left (northeast) at Granite Chief Trail junction
►8	15.0	Squaw Valley parking lot

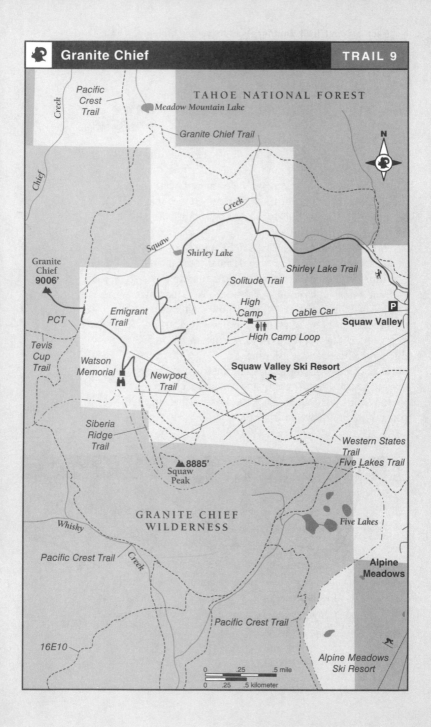

Granite Chief

TRAIL 9

TAHOE NATIONAL FOREST

Pacific Crest Trail

Creek

Meadow Mountain Lake

Granite Chief Trail

Chief

Creek

Squaw

Shirley Lake

Shirley Lake Trail

Granite Chief 9006'

Solitude Trail

PCT

Emigrant Trail

High Camp

Cable Car

Squaw Valley

Tevis Cup Trail

High Camp Loop

Watson Memorial

Squaw Valley Ski Resort

Newport Trail

Siberia Ridge Trail

Western States Trail

8885' Squaw Peak

Five Lakes Trail

GRANITE CHIEF WILDERNESS

Five Lakes

Whisky

Alpine Meadows

Creek

Pacific Crest Trail

Pacific Crest Trail

16E10

Alpine Meadows Ski Resort

0   .25   .5 mile
0   .25   .5 kilometer

Granite Chief

At 9,006 feet, Granite Chief is the centerpiece of the surrounding Granite Chief Wilderness, directly west of Squaw Valley USA. An excellent view from the summit is available from two different approaches requiring two different levels of commitment. The first alternative follows a stiff climb from Squaw Valley along Squaw Creek, past Shirley Lake, and over the Sierra Crest to the base of the peak. The second utilizes the aerial cable car from Squaw Valley to High Camp, greatly reducing the effort and time involved to reach the summit. Whichever way you choose, the view from the top is excellent and the scenery along the way is quite rewarding as well.

Best Time

Though the route is usually snow-free mid-July–mid-October, wildflowers are typically at their peak late July–mid-August.

Finding the Trail

From CA 89, about 8.5 miles south of Truckee and 5 miles north of Tahoe City, head west on Squaw Valley Road for 2.25 miles into the center of Squaw Valley. Turn right on Squaw Peak Road and continue to the lower intersection with Squaw Peak Way and park in the wide shoulder. If you opt for the cable car route, simply park in the main parking lot of Squaw Valley and take the short walk to the cable car building.

TRAIL USE
Hike

LENGTH
10.2 miles, 4–6 hours

VERTICAL FEET
±3,425

DIFFICULTY
– 1 2 3 4 **5** +

TRAIL TYPE
Out-and-back

SURFACE TYPE
Dirt, Paved

FEATURES
Canyon
Mountain
Summit
Stream
Lake
Birds
Cool & Shady
Great Views
Photo Opportunity

FACILITIES
None

High Camp offers the possibility of a high-class adventure. After the climb of Granite Chief, hikers can swim in the pool, revive at the spa, dine at one of the cafes or restaurants, or sip a cold one in the bar.

Cool & Shady

Logistics

Parking is not available at the Shirley Lake Trailhead, near the upper intersection between Squaw Peak Road and Squaw Peak Way. While taking the aerial tram up to High Camp will save 2.5 miles of hiking and nearly 2,000 feet of elevation gain, you'll have to cough up $39 for the ride. However, if you walk all the way from the bottom of Squaw Valley, you can ride the cable car from High Camp back to Squaw Valley for free.

▶1 From the parking area follow a short dirt path that leads to the actual trailhead, which is near the upper intersection of Squaw Peak Road and Squaw Peak Way. Find the continuation of the path along the left-hand bank of Squaw Creek, which is sheltered by red firs and lodgepole and Jeffrey pines. Lacking a single designated route, multiple paths follow a moderately steep course upstream past shrubs and around boulders. At some point you'll probably come to the realization that this trail evolved from repeated use and wasn't the result of a trail builder's thoughtful design. Entering a shady forest, thimbleberry and bracken fern carpet the canyon floor, while the tumbling creek drops over short rock steps and into picturesque pools.

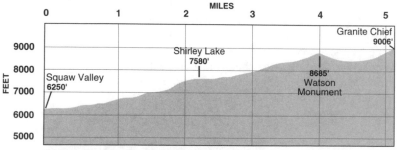

TRAIL 9 Granite Chief Elevation Profile

Squaw Valley Aerial Tram

OPTION

The Squaw Valley Aerial Tram makes it possible to opt out of ascending or descending, and shortens the length by half, to 5.0 miles, and the time to three hours.

Leave the forest cover to climb steeply over boulders and slabs, where blue paint blazes help to keep you on route. After hopping across a side stream you reenter mixed forest, as western white pines join the previously mentioned conifers. Continue the stiff climb alongside the creek, which is lined with lush vegetation and wildflowers in season. The grade temporarily abates as you reach the top of an open bench and enjoy a limited view of the surroundings before returning to a climb through the trees. Eventually the trail veers away from Squaw Creek and leads to a log crossing of an alder-lined tributary stream, 1.25 miles from the trailhead.

Beyond the stream crossing you climb over an extensive area of granite slabs and boulders with intermittent stretches of dirt trail. The open terrain allows views of the canyon and Squaw Valley below, as well as the supports and cables for the passing cable cars on your left. The grade eases a bit above the slabs and you follow a mild ascent through scattered forest and around granite humps. A short descent then leads to the shoreline of diminutive and shallow Shirley Lake, 2.2 miles from the trailhead. ▶2 Lodgepole pines and mountain hemlocks on the near shore, and meadows and shrubs on the far shore, rim the lake. An area of granite cliffs lends an alpine ambience to the lake.

The trail heads south from the lake and makes a steep climb via switchbacks under a chairlift and across wildflower-carpeted slopes to Shirley Lake Road. Proceed along this road past the junction of

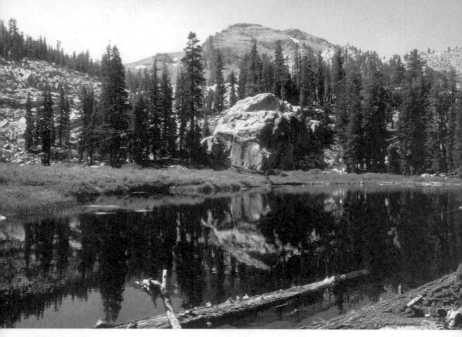

Shirley Lake

the Solitude Trail, at 2.8 miles. ►3 Continue on a steep climb, which zigzags beneath the Shirley Lake Express chairlift for 0.4 mile, to a signed junction with the High Camp Loop Trail. ►4 Those who elected to ride the cable car join the trail at this point, having walked 0.3 mile from High Camp along the north side of the loop trail.

Following signed directions toward Emigrant Peak, Siberia Ridge, and Newport; turn right on the High Camp Loop Trail; and climb along the dirt road toward the Sierra Crest. In early season the open slopes surrounding the route are extensively carpeted with mule-ears, lupine, and other wild-flowers. Soon you reach another junction, where the loop trail bends to the left but you veer to the right. ►5 Pass above the Shirley Lake Express chairlift and then below the Emigrant chairlift on the way to signed junction D. ►6

At junction D, turn right, obeying signs for Squaw Peak and Emigrant Peak, and climb a short

Wildflowers

Photo Opportunity 📷

distance to junction E. ►7 Turn right and follow the Emigrant Trail to the crest of the ridge and the site of the Watson Monument. ►8

From the monument, descend along the ridge to a saddle and a signed junction at a hairpin turn. ►9 Turn right and follow this trail for a short distance to a three-way junction with the Pacific Crest Trail (PCT). ►10 Following signed directions for Granite Chief, you veer right and climb to the crest of the east ridge of Granite Chief. ►11 Leave the PCT at the top of the ridge and follow a use trail for 0.3 mile to the summit. ►12 Views from the top of Granite Chief are quite rewarding, including the Desolation peaks to the south, Castle Peak and the terrain around Donner Pass to the north, and part of Lake Tahoe to the east.

🚶		MILESTONES
►1	0.0	Start at trailhead
►2	2.2	Shirley Lake
►3	2.8	Continue straight (southwest) ahead at Solitude Trail junction
►4	3.2	Turn right (southwest) at High Camp Loop Trail junction
►5	3.3	Continue straight ahead (southwest) at Newport junction
►6	3.7	Turn right (west) at Siberia Ridge junction
►7	3.8	Turn right (north) at Emigrant junction
►8	4.0	Watson Monument
►9	4.4	Turn right (northwest) at junction in saddle
►10	4.6	Turn right (north) at Pacific Crest Trail junction
►11	4.7	Leave PCT at southeast ridge of Granite Peak
►12	5.1	Summit of Granite Chief

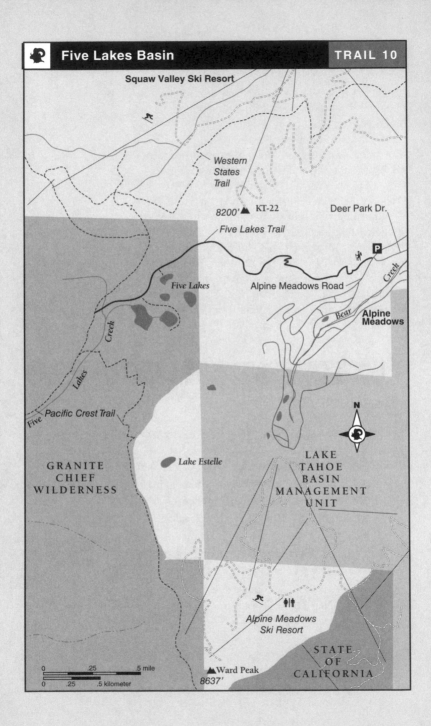

Five Lakes Basin

A short but steep climb leads to a forested basin holding five serene, forest-rimmed lakes which are well suited for an afternoon of sunbathing, picnicking, fishing, or just relaxing. Because the lakes are only an hour from the trailhead, don't expect to be alone, particularly on weekends.

Best Time

Snow leaves the trail by mid-July and usually returns after October.

Finding the Trail

Approximately 10 miles south of Truckee and 4 miles north of Tahoe City, leave CA 89 and follow Alpine Meadows Road for 2.1 miles to the trailhead, which will be on the right-hand side of the road, opposite an intersection of Deer Park Drive. Park along either shoulder of the road, as conditions allow.

Logistics

Due to overuse, camping is not allowed in the Five Lakes Basin.

Trail Description

▶1 Leave the trailhead and begin a moderate climb across shrub-covered slopes carpeted with a dense tangle of manzanita, snowberry, and huckleberry oak, and dotted with a few Jeffrey pines and white

TRAIL USE
Hike, Run,
Dogs Allowed
LENGTH
4.0 miles, 2–3 hours
Vertical feet
±1,000
DIFFICULTY
– 1 2 **3** 4 5 +
TRAIL TYPE
Out-and-back
SURFACE TYPE
Dirt

FEATURES
Canyon
Mountain
Lake
Photo Opportunity

FACILITIES
None

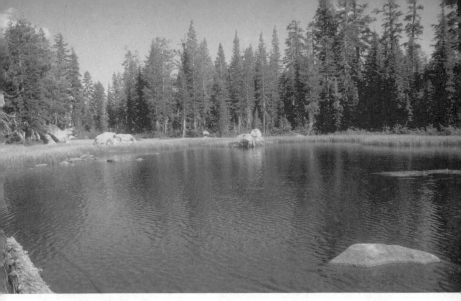

Largest *of Five Lakes*

Canyon 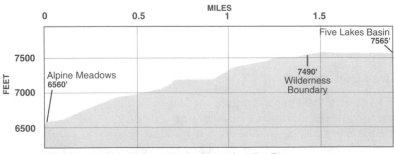 firs. Views of the canyon and the Alpine Meadows Ski Area improve with the subsequent gain in elevation, as you continue up the open, south-facing hillside. Higher up the slope a series of switchbacks leads to an arcing ascent that takes you across a granitic ridge, where stunted western white pines and Jeffrey pines eke out an existence in the inhospitable surroundings. This section of the climb feels very alpine thanks to the granitic rock and the vertical exposure. The grade momentarily eases, but all too soon you resume climbing, crossing the Granite

TRAIL 10 Five Lakes Basin Elevation Profile

Chief Wilderness boundary near a stand of red firs, 1.4 miles from the trailhead. ▶2

Past the boundary the steep climb moderates for good and you stroll through moderate forest cover, soon encountering a short use trail heading southwest to the first of the forest-rimmed lakes. A short distance farther, at 1.9 miles, is a three-way junction, where the left-hand trail heads toward the largest lake. ▶3

Easy access to the Pacific Crest Trail beyond the Five Lakes Basin provides hikers with plenty of opportunities for further wanderings.

🚶	**MILESTONES**	
▶1	0.0	Start at trailhead
▶2	1.4	Granite Chief Wilderness boundary
▶3	1.9	Junction to largest lake trail

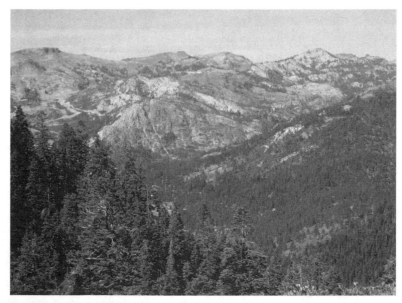

View *from Five Lakes Trail*

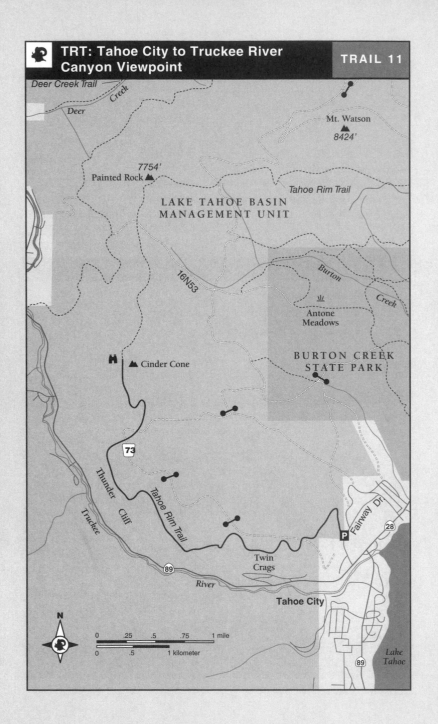

Deer Creek Trail

Deer Creek

Mt. Watson
8424'

7754'
Painted Rock

Tahoe Rim Trail

LAKE TAHOE BASIN
MANAGEMENT UNIT

16N53

Burton Creek

Antone Meadows

Cinder Cone

BURTON CREEK
STATE PARK

73

Thunder Cliff

Truckee

Tahoe Rim Trail

P

Fairway Dr

28

89

Twin Crags

River

Tahoe City

89

Lake Tahoe

N

0   .25   .5   .75   1 mile
0   .5   1 kilometer

Tahoe Rim Trail: Tahoe City to Truckee River Canyon Viewpoint

This section of the Tahoe Rim Trail climbs steeply away from the hubbub around Tahoe City to a couple of fine vista points, one of the Lake Tahoe Basin and another of the Truckee River Canyon.

Best Time

Winter snow typically disappears from this area by June. The trail remains open until the first major storm of autumn, usually sometime in late October or early November.

Finding the Trail

From the junction of CA 28 and CA 89 in Tahoe City, proceed northbound on CA 89 for 0.1 mile and turn right onto Fairway Drive. Follow Fairway for 0.25 mile to the Fairway Community Center and park in its lot. The trail begins across the street.

Trail Description

▶1 The trail attacks the steep hillside with a vengeance, switchbacking up the slope through manzanita and bitterbrush beneath a light forest of incense cedars, white firs, sugar pines, and Jeffrey pines. Gratefully, the steep climb abates soon after a series of short switchbacks and then continues at a more moderate grade, as shimmering Lake Tahoe makes brief appearances through gaps in the mixed forest. After a while the trail switchbacks, ascends to the crossing of an old logging road, and then continues to a crossing of Forest Route 73, 0.3 mile from the trailhead.

TRAIL USE
Hike, Run, Bike,
Horses, Dogs Allowed

LENGTH
11.4 miles, 5 hours

VERTICAL FEET
+1,350

DIFFICULTY
– 1 2 3 **4** 5 +

TRAIL TYPE
Out-and-back

SURFACE TYPE
Dirt

FEATURES
Great Views
Photo Opportunity
Steep

FACILITIES
None

HISTORY

Fiberboard Freeway

At one time the Fiberboard Corporation held a sizable tract of timberland in the north Tahoe area. Forest Route 73, which provides a connection between Brockway Summit and Tahoe City, is known by locals—especially mountain bikers—as the Fiberboard Freeway. In addition to its interest in forest products, the company also owned the Sierra-at-Tahoe and Northstar California ski resorts during the mid-1990s. The company divested itself of the woods products division in 1995 for the sum of $239 million.

Great Views 🔭

The Tahoe Rim Trail (TRT) continues climbing moderately through mixed forest until you reach the edge of the rim of the Truckee River Canyon above Twin Crags, about a mile from the trailhead. Here, fine views open up of Lake Tahoe and the Granlibakken ski runs across the canyon. Eventually the trail leaves the views behind, entering the forest again on an ascent over a low rise. Recent logging activity has created some unsightly areas along this stretch, but they're quickly forgotten when you come back along the edge of the canyon above Thunder Cliff. Excellent views of the Truckee River

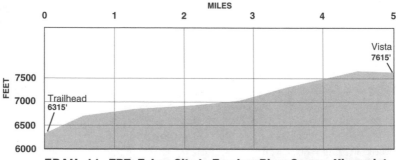

TRAIL 11   TRT: Tahoe City to Truckee River Canyon Viewpoint Elevation Profile

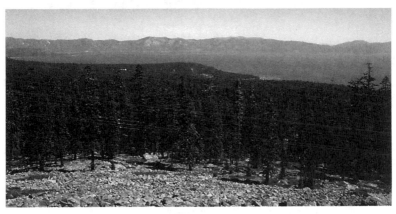

View *of Lake Tahoe from the Tahoe Rim Trail*

accompany this romp along the top of the cliff for the next 0.5 mile.

The trail veers away from the canyon edge and heads back into fir forest on a moderate, occasionally switchbacking climb. A mile or so from Thunder Cliff, the TRT traverses around the west slope of the volcanic Cinder Cone, where a grand view of the Truckee River Canyon unfolds, including Alpine Meadows, as well as a part of Lake Tahoe and Twin Peaks, a more-than-suitable reward for the 5-plus-mile climb. A short walk farther reveals a second vista point, ►2 where a piece of Squaw Valley joins the Alpine Meadows view. Plenty of rocks at both locations offer excellent perches to sit upon and enjoy the views. After thoroughly enjoying the surroundings, retrace your steps 5.7 miles to the trailhead.

Great Views

Great Views

🚶	**MILESTONES**	
►1	0.0	Start at Tahoe Rim Trailhead
►2	5.4	Cinder Cone viewpoint

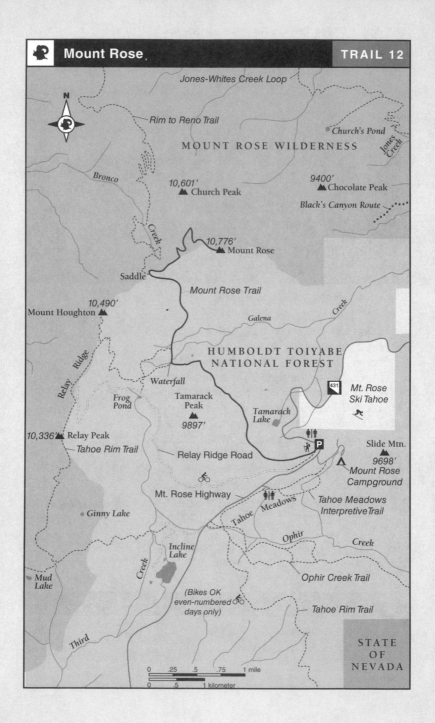

Jones-Whites Creek Loop

Rim to Reno Trail

Church's Pond

Jones Creek

MOUNT ROSE WILDERNESS

Bronco

9400'
▲ Chocolate Peak

10,601'
▲ Church Peak

Black's Canyon Route

Creek

10,776'
▲ Mount Rose

Saddle

Mount Rose Trail

10,490'
Mount Houghton ▲

Galena

Creek

HUMBOLDT TOIYABE
NATIONAL FOREST

Relay Ridge

Waterfall

431

Mt. Rose
Ski Tahoe

Frog
Pond

Tamarack
Peak
▲
9897'

Tamarack
Lake

10,336' ▲ Relay Peak

Tahoe Rim Trail

Relay Ridge Road

Slide Mtn.
▲
9698'
Mount Rose
Campground

Mt. Rose Highway

Tahoe Meadows

Tahoe Meadows
Interpretive Trail

• Ginny Lake

Ophir

Creek

Incline
Lake

Creek

Ophir Creek Trail

Mud
Lake

(Bikes OK
even-numbered
days only)

Tahoe Rim Trail

Third

STATE
OF
NEVADA

0   .25   .5   .75   1 mile

0   .5   1 kilometer

Mount Rose

The route to the summit of Mount Rose may be the most popular trail in the state of Nevada, as evidenced by the full trailhead parking lot on summer weekends. The attractions of this trip are many, including spectacular views of Lake Tahoe from the summit, a delightful display of wildflowers in the Galena Creek drainage, and a chance to scale the third-highest peak in the Tahoe Basin.

TRAIL USE
Hike, Run,
Dogs Allowed

LENGTH
10.0 miles, 6 hours

VERTICAL FEET
+2,425

DIFFICULTY
– 1 2 **3** 4 5 +

TRAIL TYPE
Out-and-back

SURFACE TYPE
Dirt

FEATURES
Mountain
Summit
Stream
Waterfall
Wildflowers
Great Views
Photo Opportunity

FACILITIES
Restrooms
Campground

Best Time

Though the trail is usually snow-free in early July, mid-July–mid-August is the best time to view the wildflower display along Galena Creek. Generally, the trail stays open through October, but autumn days may see an inversion layer over the Truckee Meadows that allows only a hazy view of Reno and Sparks.

Finding the Trail

From Reno, take I-580 south to the Mount Rose Highway (NV 431) exit, and proceed southwest to Mount Rose Summit (8,911 feet) and the trailhead parking area on the right. From Incline Village, the parking area is 8 miles northeast of the junction of NV 28 and NV 431. The old Mount Rose Trailhead is 0.3 mile southwest of the summit, where a service road heads toward Relay Ridge, a favorite route of mountain bikers.

Trail Description

▶1 From the parking lot at Mount Rose Summit, follow the trail on an ascending traverse above the Mount Rose Highway, across a sagebrush- and grass-covered hillside dotted with boulders and sprinkled with lodgepole and whitebark pines. Mule-ears and lupine add dashes of purple and yellow to the slopes in early to midsummer. As you continue the climb, the pines become even more widely scattered, which allows for fine views of the upper end of Tahoe Meadows and Lake Tahoe rimmed on the far shore by towering peaks. Eventually the trail veers away from the highway and enters light forest on the way to a saddle between Tamarack Peak on your left and Peak 9,201 on your right.

Wildflowers ❀

Beyond the saddle the gently rising trail slices across the eastern flank of Tamarack Peak, where mountain hemlocks begin to intermix with the pines. Gaps in the trees permit periodic glimpses of meadow-rimmed Tamarack Lake, 400 feet below, and the reddish-gray, volcanic summit of Mount Rose looming above the treetops.

Near the 1.5-mile mark the climbing ends and you begin a mild descent across steep slopes on the northeast side of Tamarack Peak. After the crossing of a seasonal stream, proceed across a forested bench

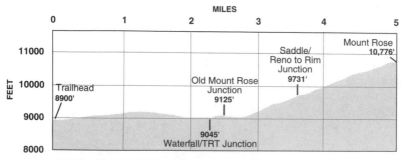

TRAIL 12 Mount Rose Elevation Profile

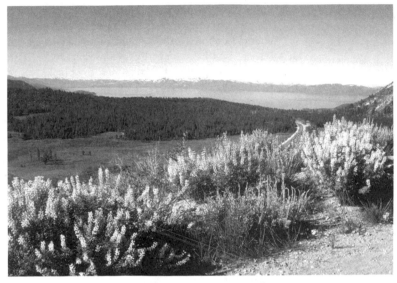

Tahoe Meadows *and Lake Tahoe from the Mount Rose Trail*

before continuing the descent across another steep hillside. Soon the pleasant sound of running water propels you onward toward a waterfall. Reaching the floor of Galena Creek Canyon, 2.3 miles from the trailhead, you come to a junction ►2 with the continuation of the Tahoe Rim Trail on the left near a waterfall. Continuing ahead, you stand below this scenic gem, where multiple ribbons of water spill picturesquely down dark rock walls. Downstream, an expansive meadow provides a fine foreground view for the massive hulk of Mount Rose.

Away from the fall, you cross the creek and skirt the base of a rock-strewn hill, opposite a willow- and flower-lined creek and lush meadow to the right. A moderate climb leads away from the creek and meadow and winds uphill to the crossing of a small tributary stream. A short walk from the stream brings you to a junction with the old section of the Mount Rose Trail, 2.5 miles from the trailhead. ►3

 Waterfall

On extremely clear days, you can see north from Mount Rose all the way to the Cascade volcanoes of Lassen Peak and Mount Shasta.

From the junction, curve around and cross another tributary of Galena Creek, where an uninterrupted climb to the summit begins. During peak season, a brilliant display of wildflowers mixes with a lush assemblage of shrubs near the creek, where the variety of flowers includes lupine, paintbrush, angelica, larkspur, and mule-ears. Leaving the luxuriant vegetation behind, the trail makes a moderate ascent of a dry hillside before turning into a narrow, steep canyon. Climb the slender cleft, twice crossing a seasonal creek, and enter Mount Rose Wilderness. At the top of the climb is a saddle amid some weather-beaten whitebark pines and the Rim to Reno Trail junction ►4, 3.6 miles from the trailhead.

Wildflowers

To reach the summit of Mount Rose, turn right at the junction and head through scattered whitebark pines along a narrow ridge toward the gray volcanic mass of Mount Rose. At the end of the ridge, the grade increases and you begin the first of five switchbacks up the west slope of the peak, where views of the surrounding countryside improve with each step. From the switchbacks, the trail makes an ascending traverse around to the northwest side of the mountain, where low-growing alpine plants soon replace the stunted pines. Another series of switchbacks climbs up the rocky slopes, while the actual summit lies just out of view. As you approach what seems to be the top, one more set of three short switchbacks brings you to the summit ridge, from where a short jaunt leads to the top. ►5

Summit

Improvements at the summit consist of a trail register and rock walls piled high to restrain the notorious winds that frequent the area. If you happen to arrive under calm conditions, count your blessings. Views are impressive in all directions. On normal days the Sierra Buttes are visible to the north, above and beyond the Little Truckee River reservoirs of Prosser, Boca, and Stampede. Lake Tahoe is the preeminent gem, encircled by an

impressive ring of peaks, including Pyramid Peak
and Mount Tallac above the southwest shore and
Jobs Peak, Jobs Sister, and Freel Peak in the Carson
Range. Reno–Sparks and the rest of the Truckee
Meadows are clearly visible from the summit as well.

大	MILESTONES	
▶1	0.0	Start at trailhead
▶2	2.3	Proceed straight ahead (north) at Tahoe Rim Trail junction
▶3	2.5	Turn right (northeast) at junction of old Mount Rose Trail
▶4	3.6	Turn right (northeast) at junction of Rim to Reno Trail
▶5	5.0	Summit of Mount Rose

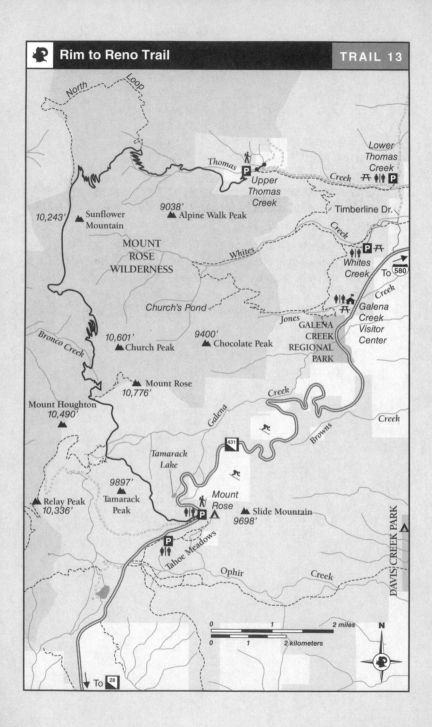

North Loop

Thomas

Lower Thomas Creek

Creek

P Upper Thomas Creek

Timberline Dr.

10,243' ▲ Sunflower Mountain

9038'
▲ Alpine Walk Peak

Creek

MOUNT ROSE WILDERNESS

Whites

P

Whites Creek

To 580

Church's Pond

Creek

Jones

GALENA CREEK REGIONAL PARK

Galena Creek Visitor Center

Bronco Creek

10,601'
▲ Church Peak

9400'
▲ Chocolate Peak

▲ Mount Rose
10,776'

Galena

Creek

Creek

Browns

Mount Houghton
10,490' ▲

Tamarack Lake

431

9897'
Relay Peak ▲ Tamarack
10,336' Peak

Mount Rose

▲ Slide Mountain
9698'

DAVIS CREEK PARK

P

Tahoe Meadows

Ophir

Creek

0   1   2 miles
0   1   2 kilometers

N

To 28

Rim to Reno Trail

At 18 miles, the newly built Rim to Reno Trail is a long hike by most standards. However, for those up to the task, the scenery is outstanding. Once past the popular Mount Rose Trail, solitude through the Mount Rose Wilderness is almost guaranteed. Seldom-seen views from the west side of the Carson Range are superb. Back on the east side, a sometimes steep drop into Thomas Creek canyon offers additional scenic delights, especially in fall when vast stands of quaking aspens turn a brilliant gold. Water is scarce away from Galena, Bronco, and Thomas Creeks, especially on the long traverse in the middle of the trip, so plan on carrying extra water.

Best Time

Snow hangs onto the upper slopes of the Mount Rose Wilderness usually through June. Mid-July–early August is oftentimes peak season for wildflowers. Snow returns to the area by mid-October in most years.

Finding the Trail

START: From Reno, take I-580 south to the Mount Rose Highway (NV 431) exit. Turn right and proceed southwest to Mount Rose Summit (8,911 feet) and turn into the large Mount Rose Trailhead parking area on the right. From Incline Village, the parking area is 8 miles northeast of the NV 28 junction.

END: From Reno, take I-580 south to the Mount Rose Highway (NV 431) exit. Turn right and proceed southwest 2 miles to Timberline Drive

TRAIL USE
Hike, Run,
Dogs Allowed

LENGTH
18.0 miles (20.8 miles),
6–9 hours (7–10 hours)

VERTICAL FEET
+2,250/-4,075

DIFFICULTY
– 1 2 3 4 **5** +

TRAIL TYPE
Point-to-point

SURFACE TYPE
Dirt

FEATURES
Canyon
Mountain
Stream
Waterfall
Autumn Colors
Wildflowers
Great Views
Photo Opportunity
Camping

FACILITIES
Restrooms
Picnic Tables

A few steps away, you stand beneath the scenic gem of the waterfall, where multiple ribbons of crystal-clear water spill picturesquely down a wall of dark rock.

on the right. Follow Timberline across a short bridge over Whites Creek and continue onto dirt surface and over a second bridge over Thomas Creek. Immediately after the second bridge, turn left onto Thomas Creek Road (Forest Route 049) and proceed 2.3 miles to a ford of Thomas Creek (high-clearance vehicle recommended). Continue another 0.3 mile on rougher road to a small parking area near a closed steel gate. There are no facilities at this trailhead.

Logistics

If you want to avoid driving your vehicle across Thomas Creek and all the way up the rough road to the ending trailhead, you can park at the lower Thomas Creek trailhead. Doing so will require hiking another 2.8 miles down Thomas Creek. To drive to the lower trailhead, simply continue ahead on Timberline Drive from the intersection of the Thomas Creek Road another 0.1 mile to a left-hand turn into the parking area. This trailhead has a vault toilet, picnic tables, and equestrian facilities.

Of course, the trail can be hiked opposite the direction described here, but doing so requires a much stiffer elevation gain.

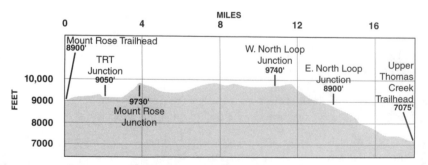

TRAIL 13 Rim to Reno Trail Elevation Profile

Trail Description

▶1 From the parking lot at Mount Rose Summit, follow the dirt trail on an ascending traverse above the
highway, across a sagebrush- and grass-covered hillside dotted with boulders and sprinkled with lodgepole and whitebark pines. Mule-ears and lupines
add dashes of yellow and purple to the slopes from
early to midsummer. As you continue the climb, the
pines become even more widely scattered, which
allows for fine views of the upper end of Tahoe
Meadows and more distant Lake Tahoe rimmed by
towering peaks. Eventually the trail veers away from
above the highway and enters light forest on the way
to a saddle between Tamarack Peak on your left and
Peak 9,201 on your right.

 Wildflowers

Beyond the saddle, the gently rising trail slices
across the eastern flank of Tamarack Peak, where
mountain hemlocks begin to intermix with the
pines. Gaps in the forest permit periodic glimpses
of meadow-rimmed Tamarack Lake, 400 feet below,
and the reddish-gray volcanic summit of Mount
Rose looming above the treetops.

Near the 1.5-mile mark, the easy climbing ends
and you begin a mild descent across steep slopes on
the northeast side of Tamarack Peak. After the crossing of a usually dry seasonal swale, proceed across a
forested bench before resuming the descent across
another steep hillside. Soon the pleasant sound of
running water propels you onward toward a waterfall. Reach the floor of Galena Creek Canyon and
a junction ▶2 between the Tahoe Rim Trail on the
left and the Mount Rose Trail ahead, 2.4 miles from
the trailhead. A few steps away you stand beneath
the scenic gem of the waterfall, where multiple ribbons of crystal-clear water spill picturesquely down
a wall of dark rock. Downstream, an expansive
meadow provides a fine foreground view for the
massive hulk of Mount Rose.

 Waterfall

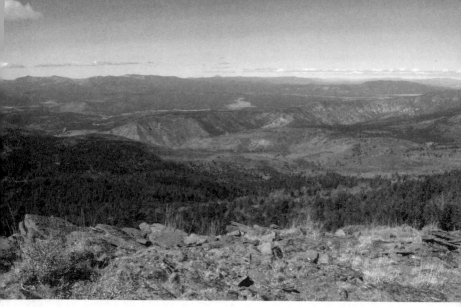

View *from the Rim to Reno Trail*

Continuing ahead on the Mount Rose Trail, you cross the creek below the waterfall and skirt the base of a rock-strewn hill, opposite a willow- and flower-lined creek and lush meadow to the right. Soon a moderate climb leads away from the creek, winding **Stream** uphill to the crossing of a small tributary stream. A short walk from there leads to a junction ▶3 with a jeep road, formerly a section of the old Mount Rose Trail, 2.6 miles from the trailhead.

Veering right at the junction, you curve around to a crossing of another Galena Creek tributary, where a stiffer climb begins. During peak season, a **Wildflowers** brilliant wildflower display mixes with a lush assemblage of shrubs near the stream, where the variety of flowers includes angelica, columbine, larkspur, lupine, mule-ears, and paintbrush. Leaving the luxuriant vegetation behind, the trail climbs moderately across a dry hillside before turning into a narrow and steep side canyon. Climb steeply up the slender defile, crossing the seasonal stream twice on the way to the Mount Rose Wilderness boundary. Amid some scattered, weather-beaten whitebark pines, you reach a junction ▶4 in a broad saddle between Mount Houghton on your left and Mount Rose on your right, 3.8 miles from the trailhead.

Continue straight ahead from the junction, dropping away from the saddle through open meadows alternating with stands of conifers. The trail switchbacks across nascent Bronco Creek a couple of times, which may be dry here in late season, before winding down the slope into light forest. The grade eventually eases and the trail heads across a perennial stretch of Bronco Creek, the only reliable source of water for the next several miles, and over to a forested flat, suitable for campsites.

Camping

Beyond the flat the trail arcs around the east side of the canyon and soon begins an extended, steady, switchbacking climb below steep, rocky cliffs to a bench directly east of Peak 9,610. The long, stiff climb is eventually rewarded by fine views down the canyon of Bronco Creek and up to Church Peak and Mount Houghton. The beautiful scenery continues for a while, as the trail follows a gentle, arcing traverse below Peak 10,083 to a forested promontory, which offers occasional viewpoints of the surrounding terrain.

The trail curves around the fringe of the promontory before turning north and embarking on a 2-mile, gently graded romp through the trees below the peaks of the Carson Range, including 10,243-foot Sunflower Mountain. Though the views are limited along this stretch of trail, the nearly level grade of the trail makes for very easy hiking. Eventually, you reach a junction ▶5 with the North Loop of the upper Thomas Creek Trail.

Turn right at the junction and follow the trail on a moderate, switchbacking, 0.5-mile climb to a saddle on the crest of the range, at 9,780 feet the high point of your journey. From the crest a scramble along the ridge to the top of either Peak 9,996 (north) or 9,890 (south) offers superb views of the surrounding terrain for anyone with the requisite energy.

Great Views

The trail drops rather steeply away from the crest into the Thomas Creek drainage (you'll more than likely be glad not to have climbed up this way), switchbacking down the steep hillside for nearly a mile before reaching a more pleasantly graded traverse across the upper canyon. The mile-long traverse eventually leads to the Thomas Creek loop junction at 13.7 miles. ▶6

Proceed along the north ridge above the canyon shortly to the top of a series of switchbacks zigzagging down the open slope toward the creek below. After reaching the canyon floor, the trail merges with a section of the old Thomas Creek Road briefly and leads to a crossing of the creek before single-track resumes. Climbing away from the creek, you proceed through a forest of Jeffrey pine, white fir, and mountain mahogany with occasional stands of aspen. After crossing an old road, you follow a set of four switchbacks down the hillside to the parking area near a closed steel gate.

Without a vehicle with adequate clearance, you must continue down the Thomas Creek Trail another 2.8 miles to the lower trailhead. ▶7

🚶	MILESTONES	
▶1	0.0	Start at Mount Rose Trailhead
▶2	2.4	Continue straight (north) at junction
▶3	2.6	Turn right (northeast) at junction of old Mount Rose Trail
▶4	3.8	Continue straight (northwest) at junction
▶5	10.7	Turn right (northeast) at junction
▶6	13.7	Turn right (southeast) at junction
▶7	18.0	End at upper Thomas Creek Trailhead

Tahoe Meadows Nature Trails

The Tahoe Meadows Interpretive Loop Trail is a wheelchair-accessible path offering a fine opportunity to experience a part of verdant, subalpine Tahoe Meadows. Not only will the wheelchair-bound enjoy this loop, but families with small children will appreciate the wide, gently graded, 1.2-mile path as well. The trail loops around the upper, northeast finger of Tahoe Meadows at 8,700 feet, exposing users to a lush meadowland environment full of verdant plants, colorful wildflowers, and trickling streams, bordered by a light forest of lodgepole pines. The Carson Range peaks of Slide Mountain and Mount Rose provide a fine backdrop to the scenery-rich meadows.

The three loops of the lower meadows offer trips of varying lengths along nascent Ophir Creek, which meanders through wildflower-covered meadows. The Middle and Lower Loops circle back to the trailhead through a scattered to light forest along a section of the Ophir Creek Trail.

Best Time

The meadows are usually snow-free by late June after winters of average snowfall, earlier in drier years. July is oftentimes peak season for wildflowers. Snow usually returns to the area by late October.

Finding the Trail

From Reno, take I-580 to the Mount Rose Highway (NV 431) exit. Turn right and proceed to the Mount Rose Summit (8,911 feet). Continue toward Incline

TRAIL USE
Hike, Run,
Handicapped
Accessible (Interpretive
Loop Trail), Dogs
Allowed (on leash),
Child Friendly

LENGTH
0.8–3.3 miles,
0.5–1.5 hours

VERTICAL FEET
Negligible to ±300

DIFFICULTY
– 1 2 3 4 5 +

TRAIL TYPE
Loop

SURFACE TYPE
Dirt

FEATURES
Mountain
Stream
Wildflowers
Birds
Wildlife
Great Views
Photo Opportunity

FACILITIES
Restrooms
Picnic Tables
Water

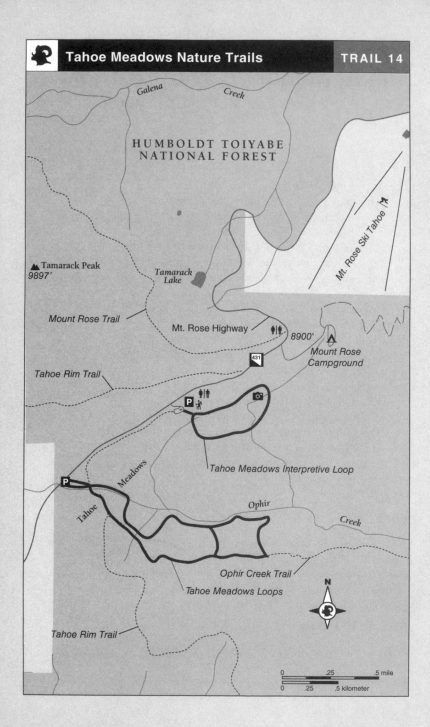

Galena   Creek

HUMBOLDT TOIYABE
NATIONAL FOREST

Mt. Rose Ski Tahoe

Tamarack Peak
9897'

Tamarack
Lake

Mount Rose Trail

Mt. Rose Highway   8900'

Mount Rose
Campground

Tahoe Rim Trail

431

P

Tahoe Meadows Interpretive Loop

P

Meadows

Ophir

Tahoe

Creek

Ophir Creek Trail

Tahoe Meadows Loops

N

Tahoe Rim Trail

0   .25   .5 mile

0   .25   .5 kilometer

Village another 0.75 mile, and turn left into the parking lot for the Interpretive Loop Trail. The lower trailhead for the Upper, Middle, and Lower Meadow Loops is another 0.6 mile down NV 431 on the east shoulder. From Incline Village, the lower trailhead is about 6.7 miles and the upper trailhead is about 7.3 miles east of the junction of NV 28 and NV 431.

The Carson Range peaks of Slide Mountain and Mount Rose provide a fine backdrop to the scenery-rich meadows.

Trail Description

INTERPRETIVE LOOP TRAIL: ►1 From the parking lot, head east on a wide, rock-lined path for 0.1 mile to the loop junction. ►2 Turn right to follow a counterclockwise circuit around the northeast, upper finger of Tahoe Meadows. Proceed across a long, boardwalk bridge over a marshy stretch of

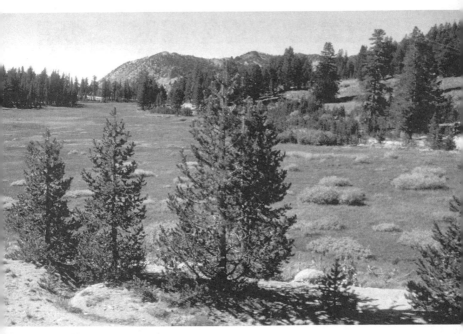

Tahoe Meadows

ground to the far edge of the meadow and then veer
northeast along the fringe, passing in and out of
shady stands of lodgepole pines.

Around the east edge of the meadow, a series of
short wood bridges takes you across boggy swales
and gurgling little tributaries of Ophir Creek. As the
loop bends back toward the trailhead, a short lateral
leads onto a low hummock of granite, from where
you have a view of the sprawling meadow from a
slightly elevated vantage. When the trail was first
constructed, this vista was more expansive, but as
the surrounding trees have matured, they have limited the view to just a sliver of the meadows. Back
on the main trail, you follow the course of the old
Mount Rose Highway along the north edge of the
meadow back to the loop junction. ▶3 From there,
make the easy climb back to the parking lot. ▶4

🚶	**MILESTONES**		
▶1	0.0	Start at trailhead	
▶2	0.1	Turn right (south) at loop junction	
▶3	1.2	Continue straight (southwest) at loop junction	
▶4	1.3	Return to trailhead	

UPPER, MIDDLE, & LOWER MEADOW LOOPS:
▶1 Descend a set of stairs away from the highway
and down to the meadows, where a short stretch of
dirt tread leads through a gap in a low fence and to
the beginning of a boardwalk. Follow the boardwalk
along the serpentine course of gurgling Ophir Creek
and come to a map showing the three loop options.
Continue ahead on the boardwalk, soon coming
to a wide deck where an inviting park bench begs
visitors to sit and enjoy the stream and the verdant surroundings. Past the bench, the boardwalk
matches the winding nature of the creek on the way
to the first junction. ▶2 Sightseers looking for just

Stream 🏞

a short, easy stroll should turn right, immediately cross Ophir Creek on a bridge, and immediately turn right again to follow the dirt path back to the edge of the highway.

Everyone else should proceed ahead on the boardwalk. After a while, the boardwalk curves right, spans the narrow creek, passes an interpretive sign, and then ends immediately before a junction with the Upper Meadow Loop. ▶3 Here the Upper Meadow Loop veers right and heads back upstream.

Taking the left-hand trail, continue ahead on the combined course of the Middle and Upper Meadow Loops. Beyond the junction the trail moves away from Ophir Creek and wanders along the edge of lodgepole pine forest above the meadows below. After 0.6 mile, you reach the junction with the Middle Meadow Loop on the right. To use this option, follow this trail south on a moderate climb for a little over 0.1 mile to a junction ▶4 with the Ophir Creek Trail and Lower Meadow Loop.

Remaining on the Lower Meadow Loop, continue ahead as the meadows narrow and the stream drops more steeply on the way toward Ophir Creek canyon. The lodgepole forest thickens a tad on the way to where the trail bends south and leaves the creek behind. Slide Mountain makes brief appearances along this stretch through gaps in the trees. Cross a seasonal stream at 1.4 miles and then make a mild to moderate climb through a mixed forest, where western white pines, white firs, and mountain hemlocks join the lodgepole pines. Reach a signed junction ▶5 with the Ophir Creek Trail at 1.7 miles.

Turn right (west) and follow the broad track of the Ophir Creek Trail, which follows the course of the old Ophir Road on a moderate climb through scattered to light forest for 0.3 mile to the junction ▶6 with the Middle Loop.

Proceed ahead on the continuation of the Ophir Creek Trail. After about 0.3 mile, the climbing ends and the trail starts a 0.25-mile descent toward the vicinity of Tahoe Meadows. Returning to lodgepole pine forest, you reach a signboard for the Ophir Creek Trail and continue on gently graded tread to a Y-junction ▶7 with the Tahoe Rim Trail angling back to the left. A short way farther is a junction with a path traveling ahead to the Mount Rose Highway.

Veer right at the junction and soon emerge from the trees to return to the lush surroundings of Tahoe Meadows. Wind around toward the bridge over Ophir Creek seen near the beginning of the hike. Here there are two options to return to your vehicle. You can cross the bridge and retrace your steps back to the trailhead ▶8 or remain on the south bank and follow the creek upstream, crossing a bridge just prior to reaching the edge of the highway, where a set of stairs leads back to the shoulder. ▶9

🚶	MILESTONES		
▶1	0.0	Start at trailhead
▶2	0.2	Continue straight (east) at junction
▶3	0.4	Continue straight/left (east) at Upper Meadow Loop junction
▶4	1.0	Continue straight (east) at Middle Meadow Loop junction
▶5	1.7	Turn right (west) at Ophir Creek Trail junction
▶6	2.0	Continue straight (west) at Middle Meadow Loop junction
▶7	2.9	Continue straight (west) at Tahoe Rim Trail junction
▶8	3.0	Turn right (northwest) at junction
▶9	3.3	Return to trailhead

Tahoe Rim Trail: Tahoe Meadows to Brockway Summit

The section of the Tahoe Rim Trail (TRT) between Tahoe Meadows and Brockway Summit was the last link of the 165-mile trail to be completed before the official opening in 2002. Offering some of the route's finest views, as well as the trail's high point atop Relay Peak (10,338 feet), one wonders how we got along without this part of the trail for so long. The 19.5-mile distance at relatively high altitude is a difficult one-day hike, but a reasonable expectation of solitude in the middle section is a fine trade-off for those who are up to the task. Backpackers will find good campsites at Gray Lake, a half mile off the TRT near the midpoint of the trip.

Best Time

Wildflowers are at their peak mid-July–mid-August, but the spectacular views are always in season during the usually snow-free months of July–October.

Finding the Trail

START: From Reno, take I-580 south to the Mount Rose Highway (NV 431) exit, and proceed southwest to Mount Rose Summit (8,911 feet) and the trailhead on the right. From Incline Village, the parking area is 8 miles northeast of the CA 28/CA 431 junction.

END: From CA 28 in Kings Beach or I-80 near Truckee, proceed on CA 267 to the Tahoe Rim Trail parking area, 0.5 mile south of Brockway Summit, and 2.8 miles from the junction with CA 28 in Kings Beach. A steep dirt road (Forest Route 16N56) on

---

TRAIL USE
Hike, Run, Bike,
Dogs Allowed

LENGTH
19.5 miles, 9 hours

VERTICAL FEET
+2,900/-4,850

DIFFICULTY
– 1 2 3 4 **5** +

TRAIL TYPE
Point-to-Point

SURFACE TYPE
Dirt, Paved

FEATURES
Mountain
Summit
Waterfall
Lake
Wildflowers
Birds
Great Views
Photo Opportunity
Camping
Secluded

FACILITIES
Restrooms
Campground

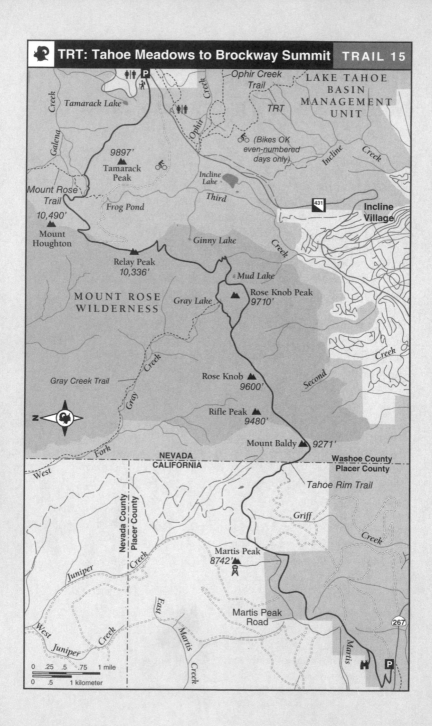

TRT: Tahoe Meadows to Brockway Summit TRAIL 15

Creek

Tamarack Lake

Galena Creek

Ophir Creek

Ophir Creek Trail

TRT

LAKE TAHOE BASIN MANAGEMENT UNIT

(Bikes OK even-numbered days only)

9897'
Tamarack Peak

Incline Lake

Third

Incline Creek

431

Incline Village

Mount Rose Trail

10,490'

Mount Houghton

Frog Pond

Ginny Lake

Creek

Relay Peak
10,336'

Mud Lake

MOUNT ROSE WILDERNESS

Gray Lake

Rose Knob Peak
9710'

Creek

Second

Gray Creek Trail

Gray Creek

Rose Knob
9600'

Fork

Rifle Peak
9480'

Mount Baldy 9271'

West

NEVADA CALIFORNIA

Washoe County Placer County

Tahoe Rim Trail

Griff Creek

Nevada County Placer County

Creek

Martis Peak
8742'

Juniper Creek

Martis Peak Road

267

West Juniper Creek

East Martis Creek

Martis Creek

0 .25 .5 .75 1 mile
0 .5 1 kilometer

P

the west side leads quickly up to a small parking area that doesn't have any facilities.

Wildflowers are at their peak mid-July–mid-August.

Trail Description

▶1 From the parking lot at Mount Rose Summit, follow new trail on an ascending traverse above the Mount Rose Highway, across a sagebrush- and grass-covered hillside dotted with boulders and sprinkled with lodgepole and whitebark pines. Mule-ears and lupine add dashes of yellow and purple to the slopes in early to midsummer. As you continue the climb, the pines become even more widely scattered, which allows for fine views of the upper end of Tahoe Meadows and Lake Tahoe rimmed on the far shore by towering peaks. Eventually the trail veers away from the highway and enters light forest on the way to a saddle between Tamarack Peak on your left and Peak 9,201 on your right.

Beyond the saddle the gently rising trail slices across the eastern flank of Tamarack Peak, where mountain hemlocks begin to intermix with the pines. Gaps in the trees permit periodic glimpses of meadow-rimmed Tamarack Lake, 400 feet below, and the reddish-gray, volcanic summit of Mount Rose looming above the treetops.

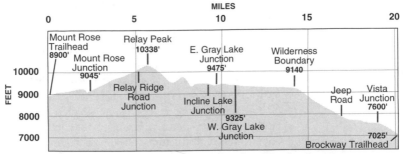

TRAIL 15 TRT: Tahoe Meadows to Brockway Summit
Elevation Profile

Near the 1.5-mile mark the climbing ends and you begin a mild descent across steep slopes on the northeast side of Tamarack Peak. After the crossing of a seasonal stream, proceed across a forested bench before continuing the descent across another steep hillside. Soon the pleasant sound of running water propels you onward toward a waterfall. Reach the floor of Galena Creek canyon and a junction ▸2 between the Tahoe Rim Trail (TRT) on the left and the Mount Rose Trail ahead, 2.3 miles from the trailhead. A few steps away you stand beneath the scenic gem of the waterfall, where multiple ribbons of crystal-clear water spill picturesquely down a wall of dark rock. Downstream, an expansive meadow provides a fine foreground view for the massive hulk of Mount Rose.

Waterfall 🏞

Turn left at the TRT junction and zigzag up the slope to the left of the cascade, soon reaching the top of the fall, where a fine view unfolds down the Galena Creek drainage. Continue climbing away from the waterfall through scattered forest to the crossing of an old jeep road. ▸3 Before the construction of the new section of the Mount Rose Trail in 2004, this rocky old road was part of the previous route to the summit.

Across the road, keep climbing through scattered lodgepole pines, passing below a power line and continuing up the slope. Farther above, whitebark pines replace the lodgepole pines of below, heralding your entry into the upper elevations of the Mount Rose Wilderness. Cross the wilderness boundary at the top of the ridge, where you encounter a junction ▸4 with the 0.3-mile lateral to 10,490-foot Mount Houghton to the north. Now on the west side of Relay Ridge, you follow an ascending traverse below the crest of Relay Ridge, which is littered with an array of communication towers and structures. Once past the man-made equipment, the trail returns to the crest of the ridge and reaches a junction ▸5 with a very short lateral over to Relay Peak Road. From there, a moderate climb leads up the steep north ridge of Relay Peak to the top. ▶6 At 10,338 feet, Relay Peak is the highest point on the entire circuit of the TRT. The stunning vista includes a good portion of Lake Tahoe Basin, Tahoe Meadows and Incline Lake below, and a piece of Washoe Lake through the gash of Ophir Creek canyon, backdropped by a parade of distant ranges extending east into the Great Basin. The Sierra Buttes dominate the northern skyline, but on clear days you may be able to make out Lassen Peak beyond, and on the clearest of days, Mount Shasta. Unfortunately, the view is not all good for keen eyes, as immediately to the northwest you may see the results of the extensive Martis Fire of 2001, which was sparked by an illegal campfire started by careless campers.

 Great Views

Away from Relay Peak, you head down the crest of the ridge for 0.5 mile, before a series of switchbacks leads down the southern flanks of the peak on a protracted descent toward a significant saddle, losing 800 vertical feet in the process. Along the way, you have excellent views of the

Upper Galena Creek *meadow*

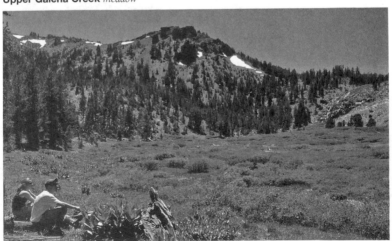

Side Trip to Gray Lake

The 0.5-mile descent to Gray Lake is a worthwhile endeavor, especially if you need a campsite. Leave the Tahoe Rim Trail (TRT) and descend away from the ridge on a section of the old Western States Trail, initially through whitebark pines and mountain hemlocks. In the midst of the descent, you cross a small, flower-filled meadow and then continue to drop through a thicker forest of lodgepole pines. After hopping across the thin ribbon of a seasonal stream, you reach the floor of the small basin and meadow-rimmed Gray Lake.

Gray Lake is a kidney bean–shaped, shallow body of water surrounded by verdant meadows. In the natural evolution of lakes and meadows, the lake is destined eventually to become a part of Gray Meadow, as it's only a matter of time before silt and debris fill the basin. On a human timetable, however, many years are left to enjoy this delightful lake. The sparkling, spring-fed water of the inlet flows down from above the lake along a rocky channel softened by rich, green moss and brilliant wildflowers. At the head of the canyon the gray, volcanic rock of Rose Knob forms a stark, contrasting background to the vibrant meadows. Over the years, numerous avalanches have swept down the side of Rose Knob, delivering an ample supply of timber to the slopes at the base of the peak.

The area around Gray Lake has limited campsites, perhaps due to lack of use despite the close proximity to the TRT. Firewood is plentiful for the time being. Swimming appears dubious, but anglers may find the fishing good.

To return to the TRT, you have the option of retracing your steps or ascending the moderately graded trail southwest from the lake to a connection with the TRT west of Rose Knob Peak, 1.2 miles from the first junction.

Donner Summit region, the seldom-traveled terrain of the West Fork Gray Creek, and, in the northwest, the trio of reservoirs on the Truckee River system and the distant plain of Sierra Valley.

More switchbacks lead to easier hiking as you approach the rocky flanks of Slab Cliffs. Nestled in the small basin below you, at the head of a branch of Third Creek, is Ginny Lake, a pleasant-looking body of water only 0.25 mile from the trail but virtually inaccessible without a steep, off-trail descent. Continuing, you pass through scattered conifers as you traverse across the rock outcrops of Slab Cliffs, with more fine views as your nearly constant companion. Away from Slab Cliffs, a lone switchback drops you into the next saddle along the ridge crest.

 Lake

A series of short switchbacks leads you down from the saddle to an unmarked junction with an unmaintained section of the old Western States Trail, where faint tread heads east to the area around Incline Lake. Just downslope, a spring near a pocket of willows provides a reliable water source for most of the summer. Remaining on the TRT, you traverse the hillside, with exquisite views of Lake Tahoe, and in 0.25 mile come directly above aptly named Mud Lake. Without a natural inlet or outlet, the brown pond of Mud Lake stagnates in its basin, progressively shrinking over the course of the summer, and in drought years disappearing altogether. Another 0.25 mile of gently graded trail brings you to yet another saddle along the crest, where nearby you'll find a junction with the old Western States Trail to Gray Lake, 9.2 miles from the Mount Rose Highway (see opposite page). ▶7

From the first junction to Gray Lake, the TRT skirts the east side of Rose Knob, where excellent Tahoe views abound. You continue to traverse the south side of the peak, through scattered hemlocks and across talus-covered slopes, before dropping to a saddle directly west of the peak, where a sprinkling of whitebark pines greets you. Heading away from the saddle, you traverse the ridge crest over to the junction with the western branch of the old Western States Trail to Gray Lake, 10.4 miles from the highway. ▶8

The traverse continues across mostly open slopes, where proclaiming the excellent views becomes almost redundant. Lake Tahoe glistens under typically sunny Sierra skies, while Incline Village, the Diamond Peak Ski Area, and the Mount Rose Highway all lie at your feet. You skirt the slopes below Rose Knob—if even grander views are desired, you can make the 300-foot climb to the top—and continue the traverse across hillsides carpeted, through midsummer, with mule-ears. Passing below unnamed Peak 9,499 and 9,271-foot Mount Baldy, you reach the Mount Rose Wilderness boundary at 12.6 miles amid scattered pines and then make a mild descent to an unceremonious crossing of the unsigned Nevada–California border.

A short zigzagging descent follows the long, open traverse, leading you down to a rock knob, from where you have another good lake view. A few switchbacks drop you past some rock cliffs to a 0.75-mile descending traverse of a northwest-trending ridge, from where you are allowed occasional vistas of Lake Tahoe and the mountainous terrain of the north Tahoe area. A scattered, mixed forest along the ridge begins to thicken toward the end of the traverse, where the trail leaves the ridge

Side Trip to Martis Peak

OPTION

For a bird's-eye view from the lookout on Martis Peak, continue on the jeep road for 0.2 mile to a junction with the paved Martis Peak Road (Forest Route 16N92B). Turn right and head uphill, following the paved road for 0.7 mile to the lookout, perched on a small flat, 0.1 mile northwest of the true summit. Along with the restored lookout, you'll find a picnic table and an outhouse. Thanks to the paved road, you may also find tourists. At one time, Martis Peak was the only staffed fire lookout in the Tahoe Basin.

to make a moderate descent to a saddle. From the saddle, a half mile of easy trail through open areas of rock, alternating with stands of forest, brings you to a jeep road. ►9 The TRT follows the course of the jeep road for about 0.4 mile before singletrack trail resumes. At this point you can make a side trip to Martis Peak (see the sidebar on the opposite page).

Leave the jeep road and descend on the single-track trail, quickly leaving the forest, to break out into a sloping meadow carpeted with mule-ears. A short way beyond the meadow, you curve around the south ridge of Martis Peak and come to a rocky viewpoint. Once again, the TRT hiker is blessed with a superb vista of the Lake Tahoe Basin. You see not only almost the entire lake but the major summits surrounding the lake as well.

 Great Views

Tearing yourself away from the beautiful view, you descend moderately back into scattered-to-light red fir forest, interrupted on occasion by yet another clearing filled with mule-ears, and farther on by a patch of head-high tobacco brush. At 2.25 miles from the Brockway Summit Trailhead, you hop over a thin ribbon of water trickling down the hillside, where wildflowers, grasses, and clumps of willow add a splash of vegetation that contrasts vividly with the otherwise dry surroundings. Beyond the thin rivulet, milder trail takes you through selectively logged forest. You then descend more moderately to the crossing of well-graded gravel FR 16N33, just 150 yards southeast of the junction with paved Martis Peak Road. After crossing the road, just over a half mile of easy hiking brings you to a junction with a spur trail to the top of Peak 7,755. ►10

A mildly graded 0.3-mile ascent up the spur trail takes you through trees and shrubs, including chin-quapin, tobacco brush, and huckleberry oak, up to a pile of rocks at the top of a hill. After the spectacular vistas previously encountered, this view seems fairly pedestrian. However, one last look at the lake may be warranted before you descend the last viewless mile of trail to the trailhead.

From the junction, 1.2 miles of hiking remain, as you follow the TRT on a moderate descent through a selectively logged forest of mainly white firs with a few Jeffrey pines. As you near the Brockway Summit Trailhead, a trio of switchbacks leads you down the hillside above CA 267, past the TRT signboard, and out FR 56 to the highway. ▶11

🚶	MILESTONES	
▶1	0.0	Start at Mount Rose Trailhead
▶2	2.3	Turn left (west) at TRT junction
▶3	3.1	Straight ahead (northwest) at jeep road
▶4	3.7	Straight ahead (southwest) at Mount Houghton junction
▶5	5.2	Straight ahead (southwest) at Relay Peak Road junction
▶6	5.7	Summit of Relay Peak
▶7	9.2	East Gray Lake junction
▶8	10.4	West Gray Lake junction
▶9	14.8	Jeep road
▶10	18.3	Viewpoint junction
▶11	19.5	End at Brockway Summit trailhead

Tahoe Rim Trail: Tahoe Meadows to Twin Lakes

Much of this section of the Tahoe Rim Trail (TRT) closely follows the crest of the Carson Range, affording travelers excellent views of the Lake Tahoe Basin to the west and the Great Basin to the east. Aside from a moderate climb from Tahoe Meadows, most of the trail follows an easy grade to Twin Lakes, a pair of shallow ponds that shrink considerably over the course of the average summer. Even considering the pleasantly graded trail, the 19-mile round-trip distance makes this suitable only for hikers in good condition. Lesser mortals can pick a shorter turn-around point and still be more than satisfied with the superb vistas. Though the largest part of this trail passes across sandy soil ill suited for wildflowers, the initial segment across Tahoe Meadows is an amateur botanist's delight.

TRAIL USE
Hike, Run, Horses, Bike (even days only), Dogs Allowed

LENGTH
19.0 miles, 10 hours

VERTICAL FEET
±3,525

DIFFICULTY
– 1 2 3 **4** 5 +

TRAIL TYPE
Out-and-back

SURFACE TYPE
Dirt

FEATURES
Mountain
Wildflowers
Birds
Great Views
Photo Opportunity
Camping

FACILITIES
Restrooms
Picnic Tables
Water

Best Time

This section of the Tahoe Rim Trail affords hikers excellent views of the Lake Tahoe Basin to the west and the Carson Valley to the east mid-July–October. Midsummer is the best time to view the flowers in Tahoe Meadows.

Finding the Trail

From Reno, take I-580 to the Mount Rose Highway (NV 431) exit, and travel southwest to the Mount Rose Summit (8,911 feet). Continue 0.7 mile to the Tahoe Rim Trailhead parking lot on the highway's south side, which has restrooms and running water.

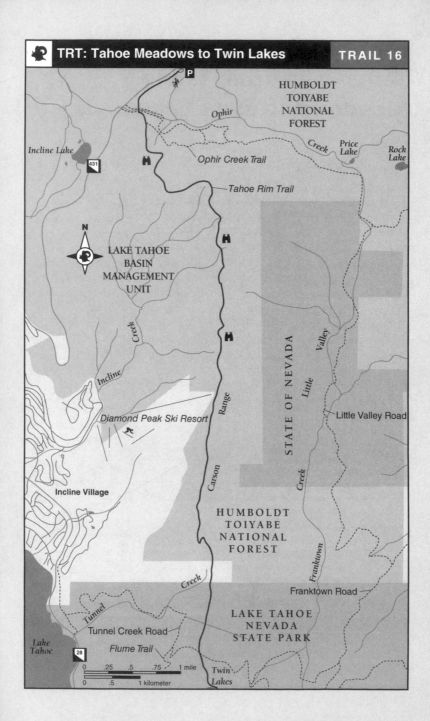

HUMBOLDT
TOIYABE
NATIONAL
FOREST

Ophir

Incline Lake

431

Ophir Creek Trail

Creek

Price
Lake

Rock
Lake

Tahoe Rim Trail

N

LAKE TAHOE
BASIN
MANAGEMENT
UNIT

Creek

STATE OF NEVADA

Valley

Little

Incline

Diamond Peak Ski Resort

Range

Little Valley Road

Incline Village

Carson

Creek

HUMBOLDT
TOIYABE
NATIONAL
FOREST

Franktown

Creek

Franktown Road

Tunnel

Creek

Tunnel Creek Road

Flume Trail

Lake
Tahoe

28

LAKE TAHOE
NEVADA
STATE PARK

Twin
Lakes

| 0 | .25 | .5 | .75 | 1 mile |

| 0 | .5 | 1 kilometer |

From Incline Village, the parking area is 7.3 miles east of the junction of NV 28 and NV 431.

Logistics

Mountain biking is allowed on this section of the Tahoe Rim Trail (TRT) from Tahoe Meadows to Tunnel Creek Road, but only on even days of the month. Hikers may want to limit their trips to the odd days, as the TRT itself and the connecting Tunnel Creek Road are very popular with the two-wheeled crowd.

Mountain Biking

Backpackers attempting the 23-mile segment of the TRT from Tahoe Meadows to Spooner Summit should be forewarned that water is at a premium along the entire route and that camping is limited to two designated sites inside Lake Tahoe Nevada State Park: Marlette Peak Campground, 13 miles south of the trailhead, and North Canyon Campground, 1.3 miles west of the TRT.

This section of the Tahoe Rim Trail affords hikers excellent views of Lake Tahoe Basin and Carson Valley.

Trail Description

▶1 Leave the TRT parking area and parallel the Mount Rose Highway as you head southwest along the fringe of verdant Tahoe Meadows, stepping across several seeps along the way. Approaching

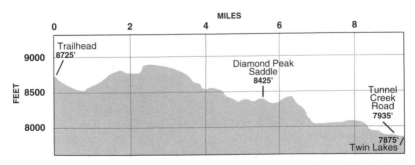

TRAIL 16 TRT: Tahoe Meadows to Twin Lakes Elevation Profile

Wildflowers 🌼 a stand of lodgepole pines near the far end of the meadows, the trail veers south across the wildflower-carpeted meadowlands to a short, wood bridge over gurgling Ophir Creek. Depending on the season, you may see the blooms of buttercup, penstemon, marsh marigold, shooting star, and elephant head among the many species of wildflower that live near the creek. Remaining on the trail to avoid damaging the sensitive flora, you continue across the meadows and into the pines, soon meeting a use trail to the Mount Rose Highway. A short distance farther, veer right (south) at a signed Y-junction with the Ophir Creek Trail, 0.8 mile from the trailhead. ▶2

From the junction you follow the TRT on a moderate climb of a forested hillside where, near the crest, you get a partial view of Lake Tahoe. Step across an old dirt road and begin a traverse of the sparsely forested slopes above the Incline Creek watershed, arcing southeast and then east around Peak 8,996. Scattered western white pines allow periodic views across the lake of the peaks and ridges lining the Sierra Crest and of additional Tahoe landmarks around the near shore. Where the sandy trail turns south again, approximately 3 miles from the trailhead, you encounter a pair of tiny rivulets, nascent tributaries of Incline Creek. ▶3 These rivulets, lined with willows, wildflowers, and young aspens, may provide the only water source along the TRT between Ophir Creek and Twin Lakes, though late in the season both the rivulets and the lakes may be dry.

Continue traversing along the west side of the ridge, below the north–south apex of the Carson Range through sparse forest, which now includes some mountain hemlocks. Following a pair of switchbacks, you follow descending trail to a prominent saddle north of Peak 8,777. Just beyond the saddle, the trail crosses to the east side of the ridge and you have your first views of Washoe Lake, Eagle Valley, and the Virginia Range.

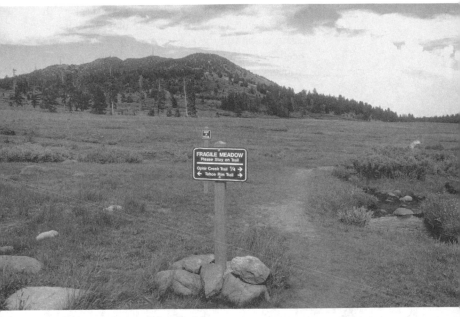

FRAGILE MEADOW sign *in Tahoe Meadows*

Follow the narrow ridge crest, with alternating views to the east and west. Near the 5-mile mark you encounter an excellent viewpoint just off the trail, where flat-topped granite boulders provide a fine perch for enjoying the Tahoe view. Away from the vista point, the trail follows the east side of the ridge into a thicker forest of western white pines and red firs. Several signs and the top of a ski lift herald your arrival at another saddle, this one above the Diamond Peak Ski Resort between Peaks 8,538 and 8,510, 5.7 miles from the trailhead. ▶4

Great Views

Leaving the saddle behind, the trail follows the west side of the ridge through scattered Jeffrey pines. In between the pines you have more excellent views of Lake Tahoe, as well as ski runs on Diamond Peak, Incline Village below, and the long ridge between Mount Baldy and Relay Peak to the north. About 1 mile from the saddle, the trail once again crosses to the east side of the ridge and proceeds through fir forest. A little over a mile farther, you begin a moderate descent, with good views to the east. Eventually the path returns to the west side of the ridge, offering a few more lake views before entering a thick forest of red and white firs. You follow a mildly undulating trail through the trees to a well-signed junction at Tunnel Creek Road, 9.2 miles from the trailhead. ▶5

Cross the road and continue along the mildly graded TRT through a scattered forest of western white pines, red and white firs, and lodgepole pines, with an understory of pinemat manzanita. At 0.3 mile from the road, you encounter the eastern Twin Lake, in a broad, shallow bowl that is rimmed by forested hills. ▶6

🚶 MILESTONES

▶1	0.0	Start at trailhead
▶2	0.8	Veer right (south) at Ophir Creek Trail junction
▶3	3±	Crossings of Incline Creek
▶4	5.7	Diamond Peak saddle
▶5	9.2	Junction of Tunnel Creek Road
▶6	9.5	Twin Lakes

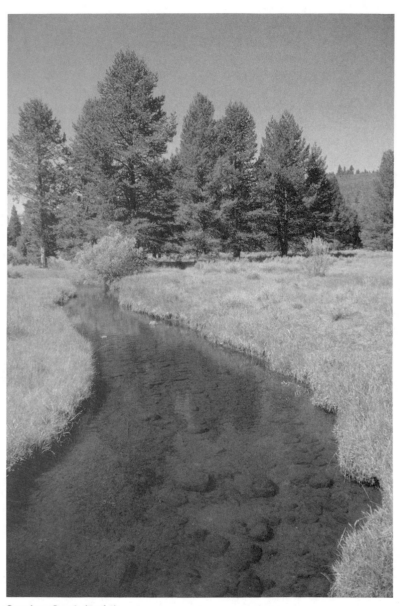

Sagehen Creek (*Trail 2*)

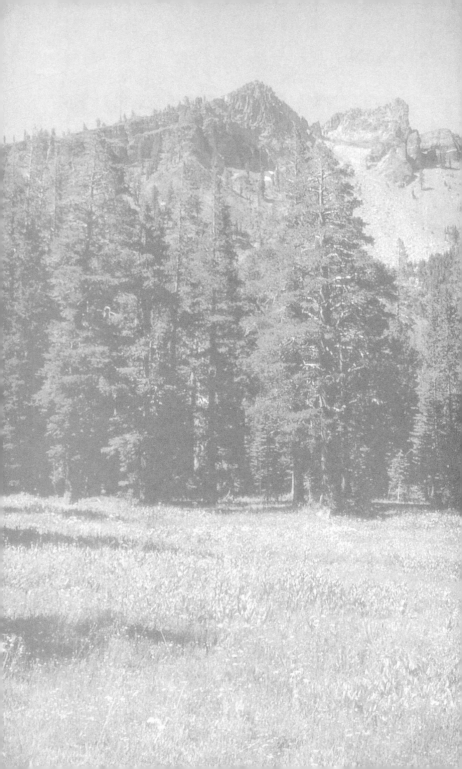

CHAPTER 2

West Tahoe

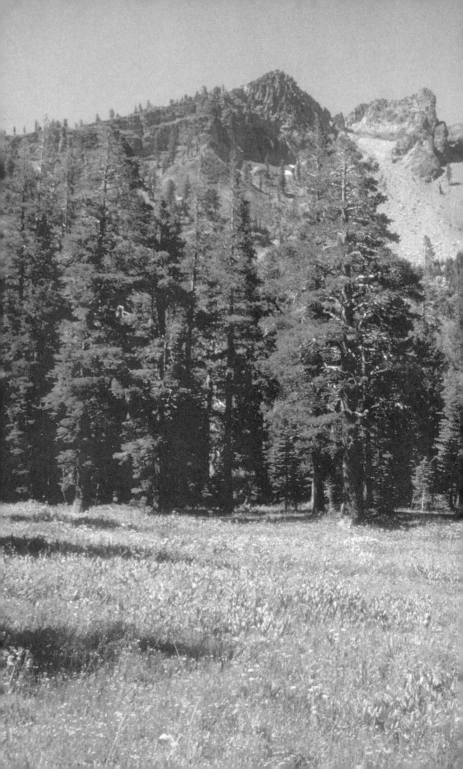

West Tahoe

S andwiched between the mega ski resorts of north Tahoe and the casinos and commercialism of south Tahoe, the west side of the lake seems relaxed and sedate. More than the other sides of the lake, the backcountry above the west shore is about walking through dense forests and strolling along peaceful streams, though the area is not entirely devoid of high summits with excellent vistas. You'll find plenty of history here, including a couple of state parks that provide glimpses into the past.

CA 89 provides the principal access to the west side of Lake Tahoe, with no other paved highways crossing the mountains between Tahoe City and South Lake Tahoe.

The Lake Tahoe Basin Management Unit oversees the national forests on the west side of the lake. Ed Z'Berg Sugar Pine Point State Park and D. L. Bliss State Park administer lakeshore units involving trails described in this chapter.

Permits and Maps

Permits are not required for either day hikes or backpacks. Entry fees are collected for state parks.

U.S. Forest Service maps covering west Tahoe are available at the Taylor Creek Visitor Center or the ranger station in Truckee. USGS maps pertaining to the trips described in this chapter are listed in Appendix 4.

Opposite and overleaf: *Twin Peaks Meadow (Trail 17)*

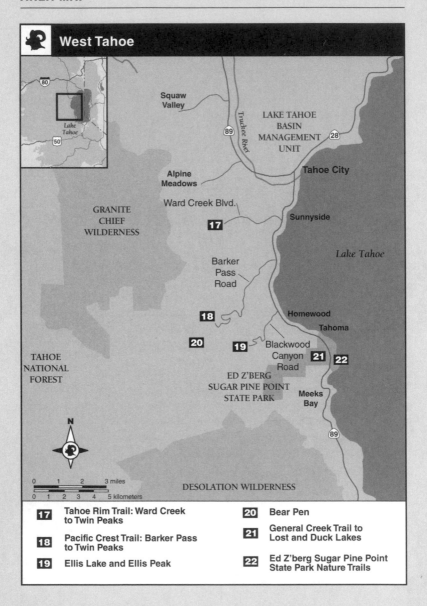

West Tahoe

Squaw Valley

LAKE TAHOE BASIN MANAGEMENT UNIT

89

28

Tahoe City

Alpine Meadows

Ward Creek Blvd.

17

GRANITE CHIEF WILDERNESS

Sunnyside

Lake Tahoe

Barker Pass Road

18

Homewood

Tahoma

20

19

Blackwood Canyon Road

21

22

TAHOE NATIONAL FOREST

ED Z'BERG SUGAR PINE POINT STATE PARK

Meeks Bay

89

N

0   1   2   3 miles

0 1 2 3 4   5 kilometers

DESOLATION WILDERNESS

17 Tahoe Rim Trail: Ward Creek to Twin Peaks	**20** Bear Pen
18 Pacific Crest Trail: Barker Pass to Twin Peaks	**21** General Creek Trail to Lost and Duck Lakes
19 Ellis Lake and Ellis Peak	**22** Ed Z'berg Sugar Pine Point State Park Nature Trails

West Tahoe Trails

TRAIL	DIFFICULTY	LENGTH	TYPE	USES & ACCESS	TERRAIN	FLORA & FAUNA	EXPOSURE & OTHER
17	3	11.6	Point-to-point	Day Hiking, Running, Mountain Biking, Horses, Dogs Allowed	Canyon, Mountain, Summit, Stream, Waterfall	Wildflowers	Great Views, Photo Opportunity
18	4	11.2	Point-to-point	Day Hiking, Running, Mountain Biking, Dogs Allowed	Mountain, Summit, Lake/Shore	Wildflowers, Birds	Great Views, Photo Opportunity
19	4	8.6	Point-to-point	Day Hiking, Running, Mountain Biking, Dogs Allowed	Mountain, Summit, Lake/Shore		Great Views, Photo Opportunity, Camping, Steep
20	4	13.4	Point-to-point	Day Hiking, Running, Horses, Child-Friendly	Canyon, Stream	Wildflowers	Camping, Secluded
21	3	13.0	Point-to-point	Day Hiking, Running, Mountain Biking, Horses, Child-Friendly	Canyon, Mountain, Stream, Lake/Shore		Cool & Shady, Great Views, Camping, Secluded
22	1	0.25–1.7	Loop	Day Hiking, Child-Friendly, Wheelchair Access	Lake/Shore	Wildflowers, Wildlife	Cool & Shady, Great Views

USES & ACCESS
- Day Hiking
- Running
- Mountain Biking
- Horses
- Dogs Allowed
- Child-Friendly
- Wheelchair Access
- Permit

TYPE
- Loop
- Out-and-back
- Point-to-point

DIFFICULTY
- 1 2 3 4 5 +
- less   more

TERRAIN
- Canyon
- Mountain
- Summit
- Stream
- Waterfall
- Lake/Shore

FLORA & FAUNA
- Autumn Colors
- Wildflowers
- Birds
- Wildlife

EXPOSURE
- Cool & Shady
- Great Views
- Photo Opportunity

OTHER
- Camping
- Secluded
- Historical Interest
- Geologic Interest
- Steep

West Tahoe

General Creek Trail to Lost and Duck Lakes .... 14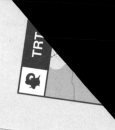
A delightful, shady streamside stroll is followed a stiff climb to a pair of secluded lakes, which m fine spots for a swim or a picnic.

Ed Z'berg Sugar Pine Point State Park Nature Trails 153
Great short trips for families and sightseers, the three nature trails within Ed Z'berg Sugar Pine Point State Park offer plenty of human history, natural history, and scenery. Swimming in the chilly waters of Lake Tahoe, picnicking along the shore, or touring one of Tahoe's old mansions—all this and more is available within this fine state park.

TRAIL 22

Hike, Child Friendly,
Handicapped
Accessible
0.25–1.7 miles,
Out-and-back or Loop
Difficulty: **1** 2 3 4 5

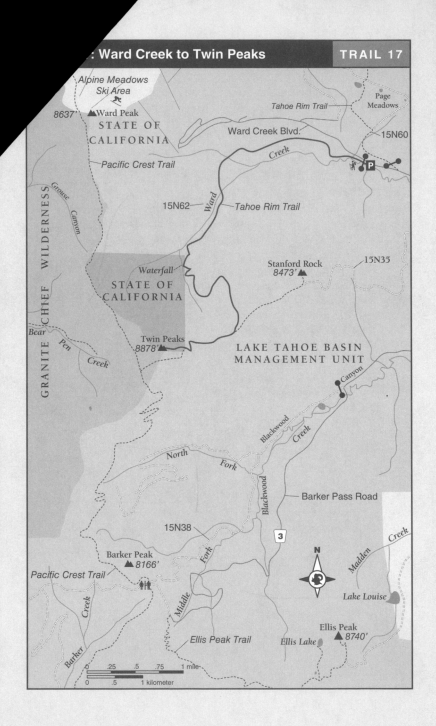

Alpine Meadows
Ski Area

Page
Meadows

8637' ▲Ward Peak

Tahoe Rim Trail

STATE OF
CALIFORNIA

Ward Creek Blvd.

15N60

Creek

Pacific Crest Trail

Ward

15N62

Tahoe Rim Trail

GRANITE CHIEF WILDERNESS

Grouse Canyon

Waterfall

Stanford Rock
8473' ▲

15N35

STATE OF
CALIFORNIA

Bear

Pen

Creek

Twin Peaks
8878' ▲

LAKE TAHOE BASIN
MANAGEMENT UNIT

Canyon

Blackwood

Creek

North

Fork

Blackwood

Barker Pass Road

15N38

3

Barker Peak
▲ 8166'

Fork

Pacific Crest Trail

N

Madden

Creek

Creek

Barker

Middle

Fork

Lake Louise

Ellis Peak Trail

Ellis Lake

Ellis Peak
▲ 8740'

0   .25   .5   .75   1 mile

0   .5   1 kilometer

Tahoe Rim Trail: Ward Creek to Twin Peaks

This trip combines one of the best wildflower displays with one of the best summit views found anywhere in the Tahoe Basin. Despite such natural beauty, the trail is not as heavily used as one would expect. Most of the route follows the well-built Tahoe Rim Trail (TRT), but the last quarter mile to the summit of east Twin Peak is a steep off-trail climb requiring a bit of scrambling.

Best Time

The spectacular wildflower display along Ward Creek peaks during July and early August, but the excellent view from the summit of Twin Peaks is fine anytime between mid-July and late October.

Finding the Trail

From CA 89 near the community of Sunnyside, turn west onto Ward Avenue and proceed along paved road for 2 miles to a small turnout on the left-hand shoulder, where the trail is marked by a small Tahoe Rim Trail signboard and a 6- by 6-inch post.

TRAIL USE
Hike, Run, Bike,
Horses, Dogs Allowed

LENGTH
11.6 miles, 6 hours

VERTICAL FEET
±2,400

DIFFICULTY
– 1 2 **3** 4 5 +

TRAIL TYPE
Out-and-back

SURFACE TYPE
Dirt

FEATURES
Canyon
Mountain
Summit
Stream
Waterfall
Wildflowers
Great Views
Photo Opportunity

FACILITIES
None

OPTION

Point-to-Point with Ellis Lake and Ellis Peak

It is possible to arrange for a shuttle and combine this trip with Ellis Lake and Ellis Peak (Trail 19) to create a point-to-point excursion.

Trail Description

Be sure to pack along a map to help you identify all the landmarks visible from Twin Peaks.

▶1 From the turnout, walk around a closed gate and follow a gently graded road through a mixed forest of firs and pines, just to the left of bubbling, meadow-lined Ward Creek. Plenty of shrubs grow beside the road, including bitterbrush, currant, manzanita, and pinemat manzanita, interspersed with verdant grasses and a wide variety of wildflowers.

After 0.5 mile the road bends slightly away from the creek and proceeds along the valley floor, offering filtered views of the peaks and ridges along the canyon rim.

Wildflowers ❁

You enter a verdant garden of wildflowers near the crossing of a tributary stream, 1.75 miles from Ward Creek Boulevard, and continue another 0.5 mile through lush meadowlands to boulder hop across the main channel of Ward Creek. Beyond the crossing, head upstream, climbing mildly alongside the dancing creek amid more lush gardens. The profusion of wildflowers you're apt to see along Ward Canyon includes aster, columbine, daisy, lupine, paintbrush, elephant head, corn lily, arnica, and mariposa lily. At its height, this is one of the best wildflower displays in the Tahoe Basin. Continuing up the canyon, you encounter a thicker, mixed forest of lodgepole pines, western white pines, red firs,

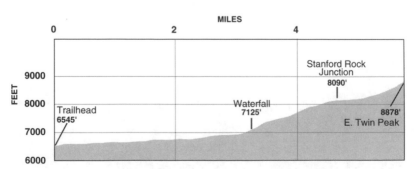

TRAIL 17   TRT: Ward Creek to Twin Peaks Elevation Profile

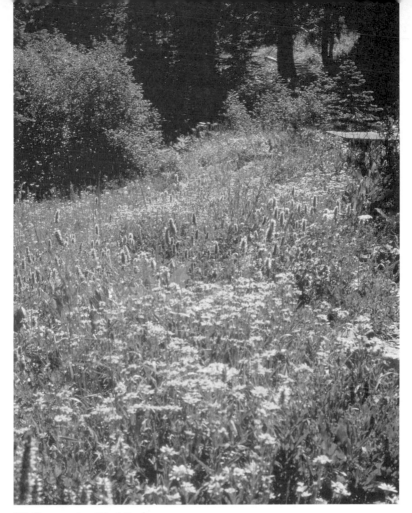

Wildflowers *along Ward Creek*

Jeffrey pines, and aspens, interspersed with pockets of lush foliage.

Eventually the trail bends away from the main channel of Ward Creek and follows a steeper route up the canyon of a side stream. Soon the sound of tumbling water heralds your approach to a 30-foot-high waterfall, 3.3 miles from the trailhead. Though the stream and fall fail to appear on the USGS map, the fall is known to locals as McLoud Falls. ▶2

 Waterfall

Continue a switchbacking climb across flower-filled slopes and pockets of light forest, with improving views of the surrounding topography. At 4.8 miles from the trailhead, you reach the crest of the ridge and encounter a signed three-way junction with a path to your left, which heads toward the summit of Stanford Rock. ►3 Peak baggers wishing to add Stanford Rock to their list of accomplishments can opt to follow this 0.9-mile one-way route to the top.

Turn right (west) at the junction and follow a rising trail along the ridge through western white pines and mountain hemlocks, with pinemat manzanita as the principal ground cover. Soon a steeper, switchbacking climb leads past a rock knob to an unmarked Y-junction at 5.5 miles. ►4 (The TRT veers left and continues on a 0.5-mile traverse below Twin Peaks to a junction with the Pacific Crest Trail.)

Summit ▲

Veer right at the junction and climb steeply up the east ridge of Twin Peaks, where you'll be treated to stunning views across wildflower-covered slopes of Lake Tahoe, the summits of Desolation Wilderness, and all the surrounding canyons. Continue the steep ascent of the ridge and scramble over rocks to the east summit of Twin Peaks and an awe-inspiring 360-degree view. ►5

🚶	**MILESTONES**	
►1	0.0	Start at trailhead
►2	3.3	McLoud Falls
►3	4.8	Turn right (east) at Stanford Rock junction
►4	5.5	Veer right at unmarked junction with use trail to summit
►5	5.8	East summit of Twin Peak

Pacific Crest Trail: Barker Pass to Twin Peaks

Follow a segment of the Pacific Crest Trail (PCT) and Tahoe Rim Trail (TRT) to the east summit of Twin Peaks, from where hikers experience a fine view of Lake Tahoe and the surrounding terrain. From an open ridge along the Sierra Crest, just before the PCT/TRT junction, you'll have additional views into the heart of Granite Chief Wilderness and the peaks of the more distant Desolation Wilderness.

Best Time

At this elevation, the trail usually is snow-free mid-July–mid-October.

Finding the Trail

Near the community of Tahoe Pines, approximately 4.3 miles south of Tahoe City, turn west from CA 89 onto Barker Pass Road (the junction is marked by signs for Sno-Park and Kaspian Campground). Follow the paved road up Blackwood Canyon for 2.3 miles and bend left at a junction with Forest Route 15N38, which continues straight ahead to an off-highway vehicle staging area. Head across a bridge over Blackwood Creek and start the long climb toward the pass on the left side of the canyon. At 4.7 miles from the creek, reach the end of paved road near the rough dirt parking area for the Ellis Peak Trailhead on the left. Continue on the well-graded dirt road another 0.4 mile to Barker Pass and the signed Pacific Crest Trail parking area on the right.

TRAIL USE
Hike, Run, Bike,
Dogs Allowed

LENGTH
11.2 miles, 8–12 hours

VERTICAL FEET
±1,300

DIFFICULTY
– 1 2 3 **4** 5 +

TRAIL TYPE
Out-and-back

SURFACE TYPE
Dirt, Paved

FEATURES
Mountain
Summit
Lake
Wildflowers
Birds
Great Views
Photo Opportunity

FACILITIES
None

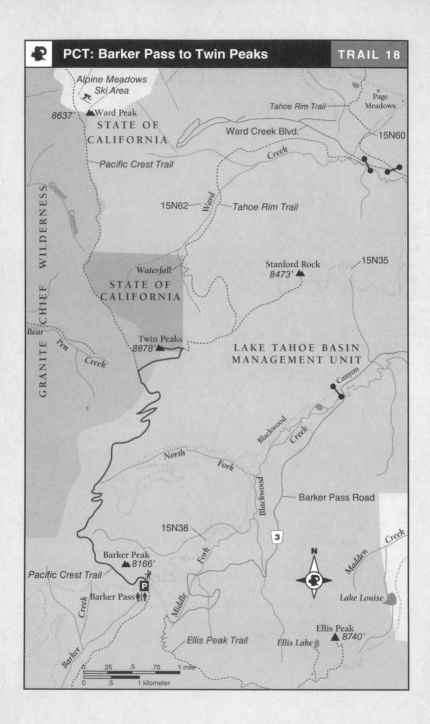

Alpine Meadows
Ski Area

8637'   ▲Ward Peak

STATE OF
CALIFORNIA

Pacific Crest Trail

Page
Meadows

Tahoe Rim Trail

Ward Creek Blvd.

15N60

Granite Canyon

Creek

Ward

15N62   Tahoe Rim Trail

GRANITE CHIEF WILDERNESS

Waterfall

STATE OF
CALIFORNIA

Stanford Rock
8473' ▲

15N35

Bear

Pen   Creek

Twin Peaks
8878' ▲▲

LAKE TAHOE BASIN
MANAGEMENT UNIT

Canyon

Blackwood   Creek

North   Fork

Blackwood

Barker Pass Road

15N38

Madden   Creek

Barker Peak
▲ 8166'

3

N

Pacific Crest Trail

Fork

Barker Pass

P

Barker   Creek

Middle   Fork

Ellis Peak Trail

Ellis Lake

Ellis Peak
▲ 8740'

Lake Louise

0   .25   .5   .75   1 mile
0   .5   1 kilometer

Trail Description

►1 Follow the wide, well-graded, and heavily used Pacific Crest Trail/Tahoe Rim Trail (PCT/TRT) through light forest around the slopes of Barker Peak, to an open hillside carpeted with scattered shrubs and mule-ears, with a fine view to the north of a pair of unnamed volcanic knobs along the Sierra Crest. You continue in and out of light forest, crossing over an old road about a mile from the trailhead. A short distance beyond the road, a path branches away from the trail and quickly leads to the edge of the ridge, from where you have a good view of Blackwood Canyon. On rising trail you head northeast to a 4- by 4-inch post below the easternmost volcanic knob, 1.7 miles from the trailhead, where a short path followed by an easy scramble leads to a partial lake view atop the knob.

Away from the knob, you drop off the ridge and follow a switchbacking 1.7-mile descent across the head of the canyon of the North Fork Blackwood Creek, through mountain hemlocks, western white pines, and red firs, crossing numerous lushly lined streams and seeps along the way.

After bottoming out, you begin a switchbacking, mile-long climb through alternating sections of light forest and shrub-covered slopes toward a rocky sub-ridge above. Approaching the crest, follow the

Be sure to pack a map to help you identify all the landmarks visible from Twin Peaks.

 Great Views

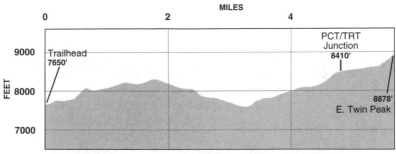

TRAIL 18 Barker Pass to Twin Peaks Elevation Profile

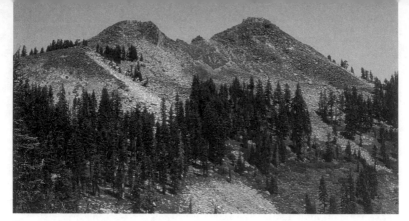

Approaching *Twin Peaks*

trail around the nose of the ridge and suddenly encounter a dramatic view of your ultimate goal, Twin Peaks. Continue climbing toward the Sierra Crest, crossing the signed boundary of Granite Chief Wilderness on the way. From the exposed ridge you have a fine view down into the canyon of Bear Pen Creek. Reach the PCT/TRT junction at 4.8 miles from the trailhead. ▶2

Turn right to follow the TRT across the south slope below Twin Peaks. After 0.5 mile you encounter an unsigned junction with a use trail to the top of the eastern peak.▶3 Veer left at the junction and climb steeply up the east ridge of Twin Peaks, **Great Views** where you'll be treated to stunning views across wildflower-covered slopes of Lake Tahoe, the summits of Desolation Wilderness, and the surrounding canyons. Continue the steep ascent of the ridge and scramble over rocks to the east summit of Twin Peaks and an awe-inspiring 360-degree view. ▶4

🚶	**MILESTONES**	
▶1	0.0	Start at trailhead
▶2	4.8	Turn right (east) at PCT/TRT junction
▶3	5.3	Veer left at unmarked junction
▶4	5.6	East summit of Twin Peaks

Ellis Lake and Ellis Peak

Ellis Lake and Ellis Peak occupy a ridgetop that lies between Blackwood and McKinney Canyons. Blackwood Canyon contains a paved road, while a major off-highway vehicle track runs through McKinney Canyon. In contrast, Ellis Lake and Peak are an island backcountry sanctuary. Though the first 0.7 mile of trail are as steep as any in the Tahoe Basin, few routes reach both a scenic lake and a 360-degree mountaintop vista in such a short distance.

Best Time

Once the snow leaves the trail in mid-July, trail users can usually enjoy the vistas from the summit or the shores of the lake until the end of October.

Finding the Trail

Near the community of Tahoe Pines, approximately 4.3 miles south of Tahoe City, turn west from CA 89 onto Barker Pass Road (the junction is marked by signs for Sno-Park and Kaspian Campground). Follow paved road up Blackwood Canyon for 2.3 miles and bend left at a junction with Forest Route 15N38, which continues straight ahead to an off-highway vehicle staging area. Head across a bridge over Blackwood Creek and start the long climb toward the pass on the left side of the canyon. At 4.7 miles from the creek and 0.4 mile before Barker Pass, reach the end of paved road and, on the left, find the rough dirt parking area for the Ellis Peak Trailhead.

TRAIL USE
Hike, Run, Bike,
Dogs Allowed

LENGTH
8.6 miles, 5 hours

VERTICAL FEET
+1,475/-425

DIFFICULTY
– 1 2 3 **4** 5 +

TRAIL TYPE
Out-and-back

SURFACE TYPE
Dirt

FEATURES
Mountain
Summit
Lake
Great Views
Photo Opportunity
Camping
Steep

FACILITIES
None

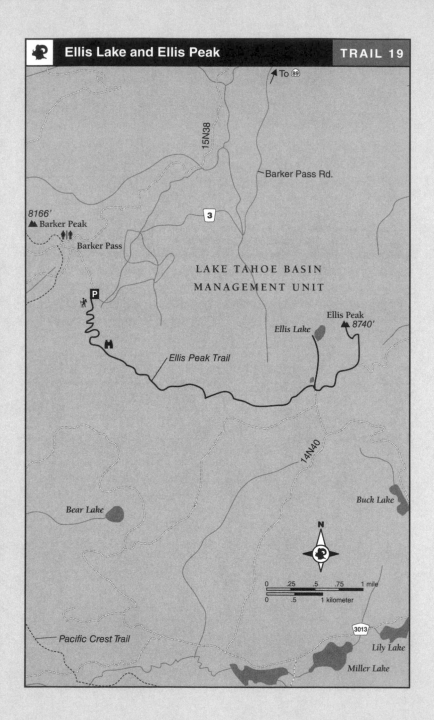

To 89

15N38

Barker Pass Rd.

8166'
Barker Peak

Barker Pass

3

LAKE TAHOE BASIN
MANAGEMENT UNIT

P

Ellis Lake

Ellis Peak
8740'

Ellis Peak Trail

14N40

Buck Lake

Bear Lake

N

0   .25   .5   .75   1 mile
0   .5   1 kilometer

3013

Pacific Crest Trail

Lily Lake

Miller Lake

Trail Description

▶1 In a take-no-prisoners fashion, the Ellis Peak Trail starts climbing steeply right from the start, as you follow stiff, winding trail up the red fir– and lodgepole pine–forested hillside. If you survive the first 0.7 mile, the grade becomes less sadistic at the crest of an open ridge, where good views of Desolation Wilderness, Twin Peaks, and Blackwood Canyon will cheer you while you attempt to catch your breath.

Leaving the switchbacks and the forest behind, you make a less intimidating ascent along the crest of the ridge through very widely scattered, wind-beaten pines and a mixture of shrubs, including bitterbrush, sagebrush, and tobacco brush. In midsummer, mule-ears and lupine add splashes of color to the desertlike slopes. Ascend the ridge for 0.5 mile, before leaving the ridge and the views behind on a 0.75-mile descent through a forest of firs, lodgepole pines, and mountain hemlocks, reaching a small meadow in a broad saddle near the 2-mile mark.

A gently graded section of old road leads away from the saddle and across slopes that were selectively logged at some time in the past. Just before the road becomes steeper, you reach an unmarked junction with a faint path, on your left. Make the

Ellis Lake and Peak are an island backcountry sanctuary.

 Steep

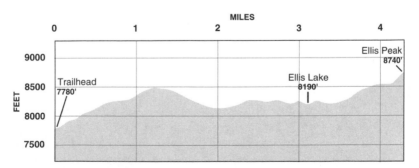

TRAIL 19 Ellis Lake & Ellis Peak Elevation Profile

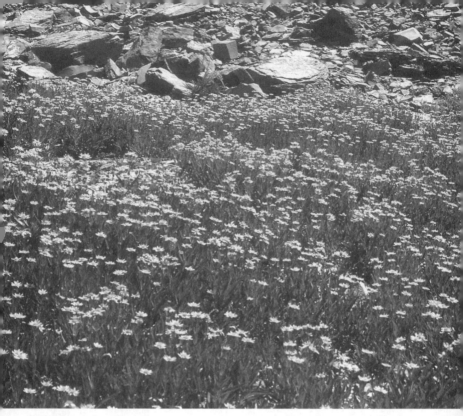

Wildflowers *near Ellis Lake*

short and steep climb up the road to a signed junction, 2.7 miles from the trailhead. ►2

To reach Ellis Lake, turn left (north) at the junction and follow the road on a mild descent through the trees. After 0.4 mile you reach the southwest shore of the forest-rimmed lake, which is nicely backdropped by the rugged cliffs of Ellis Peak. ►3 A few passable campsites can be found scattered around the lake.

Camping ▲

To reach Ellis Peak, follow the singletrack trail that climbs steeply up the hillside from the junction. ►4 After 0.3 mile, the trail merges with the road again (the right-hand road at the junction) and you continue climbing toward the summit, which has recently come into view. The road rises steeply toward the base of the summit rocks, but watch carefully for a cairn marking a section of faint singletrack trail that ascends the right-hand side of the peak to the far end of the ridge at the summit of Ellis Peak. ►5 From the summit you have a commanding view of Lake Tahoe to the east and the peaks of Desolation Wilderness to the southwest. Straight down the steep cliffs on the west face of the peak is shimmering Ellis Lake, and across the deep cleft of Blackwood Canyon is Twin Peaks.

 Summit

		MILESTONES
►1	0.0	Start at trailhead
►2	2.7	Turn left (north) at junction for Ellis Lake
►3	3.1	Ellis Lake
►4	3.5	Return to junction and turn left (northeast) for Ellis Peak
►5	4.3	Summit of Ellis Peak

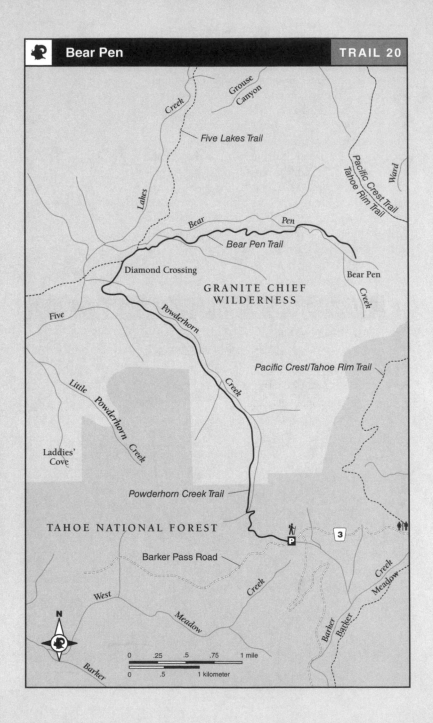

Bear Pen

TRAIL 20

Grouse Canyon

Creek

Five Lakes Trail

Pacific Crest Trail
Tahoe Rim Trail

Ward

Lakes

Bear   Pen

Bear Pen Trail

Diamond Crossing

GRANITE CHIEF
WILDERNESS

Bear Pen
Creek

Five

Powderhorn

Pacific Crest/Tahoe Rim Trail

Little Powderhorn Creek

Creek

Laddies' Cove

Powderhorn Creek Trail

TAHOE NATIONAL FOREST

P

3

Barker Pass Road

West Meadow

Creek

Creek Meadow

Barker

Barker

N

Barker

| 0 | .25 | .5 | .75 | 1 mile |

| 0 | .5 | 1 kilometer |

Bear Pen

A lightly used pocket of the Granite Chief Wilderness offers fine scenery and a healthy dose of peace and serenity. While daily quotas and fees are the rule of thumb in nearby Desolation Wilderness, a permit is not even required for overnighters in Granite Chief.

Best Time

Though mosquitoes can be problematic in midsummer, the wildflowers put on quite a floral display in mid-July. Snow-free conditions usually occur here early July–late October.

Finding the Trail

From CA 89, about 4.25 miles south of the junction of CA 28 in Tahoe City, turn west onto Barker Pass Road (Forest Route 03), signed SNO-PARK AND KASPIAN CAMPGROUND. Follow paved Barker Pass Road along the north side of the valley, bend left to cross Blackwood Creek near the 2-mile mark, and continue up the south side of the canyon on dirt road past the Pacific Crest Trail parking area near Barker Pass, 7 miles from CA 89. Descend from Barker Pass another 1.5 miles to the signed Powderhorn Trailhead on the right-hand side of the road, where very limited parking is available for two or three vehicles.

Logistics

Trails in Granite Chief Wilderness are lightly used and seldom maintained. Make sure you

TRAIL USE
Hike, Run, Horses,
Dogs Allowed

LENGTH
13.4 miles, 7 hours

VERTICAL FEET
+1,650/-1,775

DIFFICULTY
– 1 2 3 **4** 5 +

TRAIL TYPE
Out-and-back

SURFACE TYPE
Dirt

FEATURES
Canyon
Stream
Wildflowers
Camping
Secluded

FACILITIES
None

are competent at backcountry navigation before embarking on this trip, as some stretches of the trail may be indistinct.

Trail Description

▶1 Make a short climb away from the trailhead through selectively logged fir forest to a dirt road, then follow this road shortly to a bend, where the marked route continues ahead. Descend an old roadbed to a sharp curve, where you're directed by a trail marker to veer left onto singletrack trail. A steep, winding descent leads across a flower-lined stream to yet another dirt road, which is briefly followed to the resumption of singletrack trail.

Continue descending into the signed GRANITE CHIEF WILDERNESS and down Powderhorn Creek canyon. Along the descent, avalanche swaths have cleared the forest in spots and allowed a profusion of wildflowers, plants, and shrubs to flourish. Amid a thickening forest, cross a narrow stream flowing through a tangle of alders and colorful flowers and proceed on a mild to moderate descent down the canyon. The grade eventually eases where the path bisects a flower-carpeted meadow and then reaches

Wildflowers

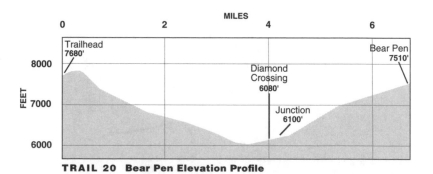

TRAIL 20 Bear Pen Elevation Profile

a boulder hop of Powderhorn Creek (early-season hikers may find this crossing to be much more than a simple boulder hop). Near the crossing is a marginal campsite.

Heading northeast, the trail proceeds away from the crossing through forest for approximately 300 yards to an open meadow known as Diamond Crossing. Pass by a marked three-way junction in the meadow, ►2 where very faint tread heads southwest to a trailhead near Hell Hole Reservoir. Continue through the meadow and then reenter forest cover on the way to a second junction, with slightly more distinct tread heading up the canyon of Bear Pen Creek. ►3

Turn right and head east on the Bear Pen Creek Trail on a moderate climb up the densely forested canyon. The trail is infrequently used and the tread tends to falter where the path crosses a small meadow. After 2.75 miles of mostly forested hiking from the junction, you emerge onto the willow- and grass-filled meadow known as Bear Pen, ►4 a large clearing lined with thick forest and backdropped by a rugged amphitheater of granite cliffs. Seldom-used, hemlock-shaded campsites scattered around the perimeter of the meadow offer secluded camping for solitude seekers. With a little bit of luck, visitors may even see a namesake critter.

 Camping

		MILESTONES
►1	0.0	Start at trailhead
►2	4.0	Proceed ahead (north) at Diamond Crossing junction
►3	4.2	Turn right (west) at Bear Pen Creek junction
►4	6.7	Bear Pen

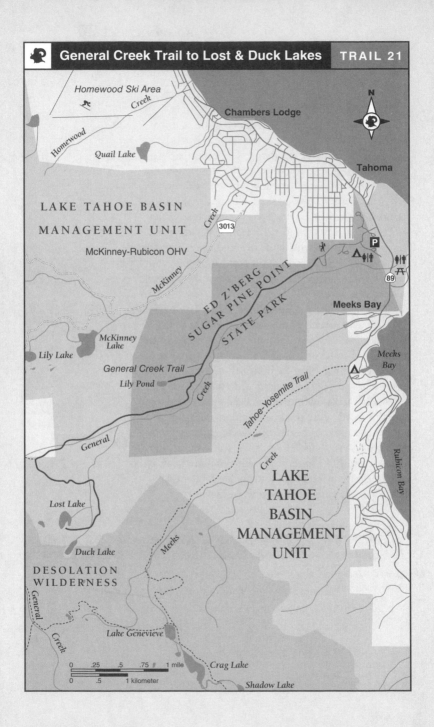

General Creek Trail to Lost & Duck Lakes — TRAIL 21

Homewood Ski Area

Homewood Creek

Quail Lake

Chambers Lodge

N

Tahoma

LAKE TAHOE BASIN
MANAGEMENT UNIT

McKinney-Rubicon OHV

3013

Creek

McKinney

ED Z'BERG SUGAR PINE POINT STATE PARK

Meeks Bay

89

McKinney Lake

Lily Lake

Meeks Bay

General Creek Trail

Lily Pond

Creek

Tahoe-Yosemite Trail

General

Creek

LAKE
TAHOE
BASIN
MANAGEMENT
UNIT

Rubicon Bay

Lost Lake

Meeks

Duck Lake

DESOLATION
WILDERNESS

General

Creek

Lake Genevieve

0   .25   .5   .75   1 mile
0   .5   1 kilometer

Crag Lake

Shadow Lake

General Creek Trail to Lost and Duck Lakes

These two quiet lakes are far enough off the beaten path to ensure a peaceful visit for those in search of some serenity. The first 2.75 miles follow a cool and shady course up the wide, forested valley of General Creek, gaining only 200 feet of elevation along the way to the Lily Pond junction. A short climb beyond the junction to Lily Pond leads to a good turnaround point for groups with young children, or anyone else looking for a relaxing stroll. Past the junction, the General Creek Trail climbs more steeply before reaching the lakes, which provide refreshing swimming opportunities.

Best Time

The trip along General Creek can be done as early as June in average years, but you'll have to wait until mid-July for the lakes trail to be snow-free. Mid-October is generally the best time to view the vivid autumn colors along the creek, before the first snowfall blankets the area in November.

Finding the Trail

Drive CA 89 to the west entrance into Ed Z'Berg Sugar Pine Point State Park, approximately 9 miles south of Tahoe City and 18 miles north of the junction of US 50 and CA 89 in South Lake Tahoe. Following signs for General Creek Campground, head past the entrance station (fee required), and continue to the day-use parking lot.

TRAIL USE
Hike, Run, Bike, Horses, Child Friendly

LENGTH
13.0 miles, 7 hours

VERTICAL FEET
±1,600

DIFFICULTY
– 1 2 **3** 4 5 +

TRAIL TYPE
Out-and-back

SURFACE TYPE
Dirt

FEATURES
Canyon
Mountain
Stream
Lake
Cool & Shady
Great Views
Camping
Secluded

FACILITIES
Visitor Center
Restrooms
Picnic Tables
Water
Phone

Trail Description

These two quiet lakes are far enough off the beaten path to ensure a peaceful visit for those in search of some serenity.

▶1 From the day-use parking area, follow paved paths to the end of the campground and the start of the North Fire Road near campsite 150. Head southwest on the wide dirt track of the old road on a gentle grade amid shady, mixed forest of red and white firs, Jeffrey pines, incense cedars, and—the park's namesake trees—sugar pines. Eventually you find yourself on a singletrack trail that makes a virtually imperceptible climb up the broad floor of the canyon, a good distance away from the placid, meandering creek and bordering meadowlands. Continue the gentle stroll through the serenity of a dense forest. Beyond a bridge over a diminutive side stream, you reach a junction marked by a 4- by 4-inch post, 2.75 miles from the parking lot, where the right-hand path follows a short climb to Lily Pond (bikes are prohibited). ▶2 Though not the most scenic body of water on this trip, shallow Lily Pond provides amateur botanists with a few interesting plant species, including pond lilies and bulrushes.

To continue to Lost and Duck Lakes, veer left at the Lily Pond junction and continue upstream along the General Creek Trail, through dense forest

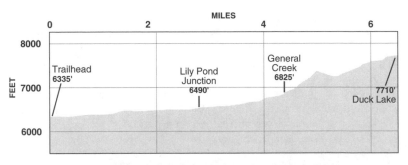

**TRAIL 21 General Creek Trail to Lost & Duck Lakes
Elevation Profile**

and lush trailside plants. Eventually the gentle terrain comes to an end where the canyon walls narrow and the grade increases, forcing the trail away from the valley floor on a moderate climb across the right-hand side of the gorge. The steady climb is briefly interrupted at a 4- by 4-inch post, where, following signage for Lost Lake, you turn left and drop to a crossing of General Creek, at 4.4 miles from the trailhead. ▶3 Short cascades drop into lovely pools along this section of the creek,

Lily Pond is a good destination for those interested in a short, easy hike.

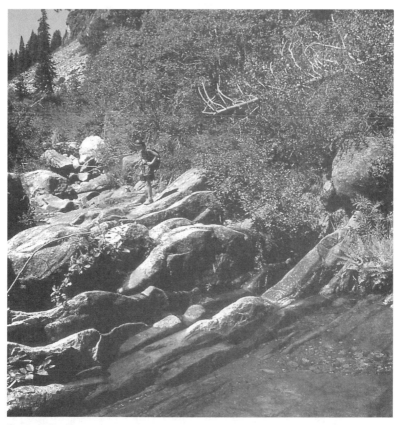

General Creek

providing a fine opportunity for a rest stop, lunch break, or perhaps a refreshing dip.

Beyond the creek crossing, make a 0.3-mile climb over granite slabs and around granite humps and boulders to a T-junction marked with a 6- by 6-inch post. ►4 Following signed directions for Lost Lake, you turn left and proceed on the wide track of an old dirt road on a short, steep climb to the crest of a minor ridge. A forested descent from the ridge offers a brief respite from the laborious ascent, beneath the shade of lodgepole pines and firs. All too soon you start climbing again on rocky road. After awhile, a thick tangle of alders, grasses, and wildflowers heralds your arrival at a crossing of the creek draining Lost and Duck Lakes, 5.5 miles from the trailhead. Continue climbing for another 0.6 mile to a second crossing of the creek. Here the road bends west and follows a gentle 0.4-mile course to a peninsula at the south shore of forest-rimmed Lost Lake. ►5 Though no defined path exists, Duck Lake is an easy 250-yard trek south from Lost Lake.

 Stream

	MILESTONES	
►1	0.0	Start at trailhead
►2	2.75	Veer left (south) at Lily Pond junction
►3	4.4	Turn left (south) and cross General Creek
►4	4.7	Turn left (east) at junction
►5	6.5	Lost Lake

Ed Z'berg Sugar Pine Point State Park Nature Trails

Ed Z'berg Sugar Pine Point State Park has a trio of easy nature trails that are sure to please the most discriminating sightseer. History abounds on the quarter-mile Lakefront Interpretive Trail, including one of Tahoe's splendid architectural wonders, the Hellman–Ehrman Mansion. The Rod Beaudry Trail provides a connection between the mansion grounds and the General Creek Campground through the Edwin L. Z'berg Natural Preserve. The 1.7-mile loop along the Dolder Nature Trail offers a serene stroll past a sandy beach with beautiful lake views to the Sugar Pine Point Lighthouse, and a return through quiet forest to the day-use parking area. Be sure to pack a lunch to enjoy at any of the several excellent picnic spots sprinkled around the park.

Best Time

Expect to find conditions good May–November on these short lakeshore trails. Tours of the Hellman–Ehrman Mansion are conducted twice daily from July to Labor Day.

TRAIL USE
Hike, Child Friendly, Handicapped Accessible

LENGTH*

VERTICAL FEET*

DIFFICULTY*

*See table below

TRAIL TYPE
Out-and-back or Loop

SURFACE TYPE
Paved, Dirt

FEATURES
Shore
Wildflowers
Wildlife
Cool & Shady
Great Views

FACILITIES
Restrooms
Picnic Tables
Water
Visitor Center

🚶 DESTINATIONS	LENGTH	VERTICAL FEET	DIFFICULTY
LAKEFRONT INTERPRETIVE TR.	0.25 mile, 15 minutes	negligible	– **1** 2 3 4 5 +
ROD BEAUDRY TRAIL	1.0 mile, 0.5 hour	negligible	– **1** 2 3 4 5 +
DOLDER NATURE TRAIL	1.7 miles, 1 hour	negligible	– **1** 2 3 4 5 +

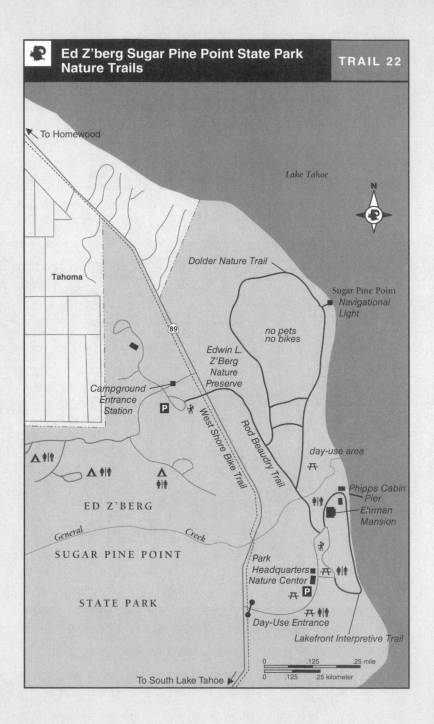

To Homewood

Lake Tahoe

N

Dolder Nature Trail

Sugar Pine Point
Navigational
Light

Tahoma

no pets
no bikes

89

Edwin L.
Z'Berg
Nature
Preserve

Campground
Entrance
Station

P

West Shore Bike Trail

Rod Beaudry Trail

day-use area

Phipps Cabin
Pier
Ehrman
Mansion

ED Z'BERG

General   Creek

SUGAR PINE POINT

Park
Headquarters
Nature Center

P

STATE PARK

Day-Use Entrance

Lakefront Interpretive Trail

0   .125   .25 mile

0   .125   .25 kilometer

To South Lake Tahoe

Finding the Trail

Drive CA 89 to the east entrance into Ed Z'Berg Sugar Pine Point State Park, approximately 10 miles south of Tahoe City and 17 miles north of the junction of US 50 and CA 89 in South Lake Tahoe. Follow the short access road to the day-use parking lot (fee required) near the Nature Center and the Hellman–Ehrman Mansion.

History abounds on the 0.25-mile Lakefront Interpretive Trail.

Trail Description

LAKEFRONT INTERPRETIVE TRAIL: From the day-use parking lot, acquire a printed guide from the Nature Center (and tickets for the mansion tour, if you are so inclined) and then wander down a dirt road toward the shoreline of Lake Tahoe to the start of the paved Lakefront Interpretive Trail. Begin your stroll near the South Boathouse and proceed northbound along the picturesque shore. You have excellent views across the sapphire-blue waters of the lake to a number of significant Tahoe landmarks, including several Carson Range peaks above the far shore. Picnic tables and park benches invite you to relax, linger, and enjoy the scenery.

 Beach

Nearing the end of the 0.25-mile trail, you pass below the expansive manicured lawn rising up to the striking Hellman–Ehrman Mansion, also known as Pine Lodge. The mansion was built in 1903 and was sold to California State Parks in 1965. The Lakefront Interpretive Trail ends near a cluster of buildings at the north end. From there you can retrace your steps to the parking lot, or follow the road behind the mansion and past the Nature Center to the day-use area.

ROD BEAUDRY TRAIL: From the day-use parking lot, follow paved road past the Nature Center and tennis courts to the beginning of the trail near the public restroom building. Turn left, leave the mansion grounds, and follow a paved path on a

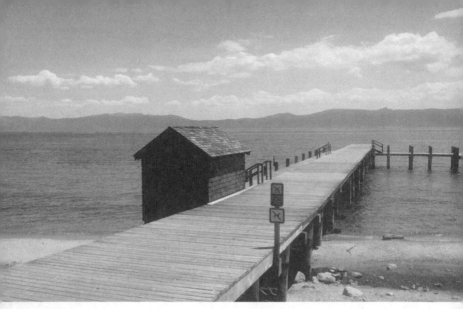

Ehrman *boat dock*

short descent to a wood bridge over lushly lined General Creek. Beyond the bridge you enter the Edwin L. Z'berg Natural Preserve, named for a California legislator who championed many environmental protections for Lake Tahoe in the 1960s. Reach a Y-junction just beyond the bridge, where the dirt path of the Dolder Nature Trail veers left.

Continue on paved trail, passing through mixed forest typical of the west shore, including incense cedars, red and white firs, Jeffrey pines, and an occasional sugar pine. Soon a grassy clearing appears, which allows filtered glimpses of Lake Tahoe through the trees on the far side of the clearing. After a short while, you reach another junction with a dirt path that provides an alternate connection to the Dolder Nature Trail and, in the opposite direction, access to a small stretch of beach. Back in forest, a mildly rising climb leads to a crossing of CA 89 and the bike path just beyond the far shoulder. A short walk from there brings you to the day-use parking lot near General Creek Campground. Without arrangements for pickup, you'll have to retrace your steps to the day-use parking area near the Nature Center.

DOLDER NATURE TRAIL: ▶1 From the day-use parking lot, follow the Rod Beaudry Trail, described previously, to the junction with the Dolder Nature Trail (bicycles and dogs are not permitted). ▶2

Head north on a dirt, singletrack trail through light forest and verdant ground cover to a grassy clearing, which, in summer, is sprinkled with lupine and penstemon. Veering toward the lakeshore, you cross a couple of connecting trails that provide access from the Rod Beaudry Trail to a section of sandy beach and a fine lake view. Back into forest, parallel the now rocky shoreline of Lake Tahoe until reaching a three-way junction, 0.6 mile from the day-use parking lot. ▶3 A short walk down the path toward the lake leads to the Sugar Pine Point Lighthouse, which in modern times is simply a blinking light atop a steel pole, mounted on a wood deck supported by four concrete pillars. Though less than noteworthy in appearance, the 6,200-foot elevation makes this the world's highest operational navigational light.

 Great Views

Back on the main trail, you continue the secluded forest stroll, eventually arcing away from the shoreline and following a mildly rising trail toward the trailhead. Ignore a couple of little-used paths from the General Creek Campground and proceed to a junction in a clearing. ▶4 A right turn will get you to the Rod Beaudry Trail, while a left turn connects to the beginning section of the Dolder Nature Trail. You can return to the day-use parking area via either trail. ▶5

🚶 MILESTONES

▶1	0.0	Start at day-use parking lot
▶2	0.15	Veer right at junction with Dolder Nature Trail
▶3	0.6	Junction with trail to lighthouse
▶4	1.5	Junction with return trails
▶5	1.7	Return to day-use parking lot

CHAPTER 3

South Tahoe

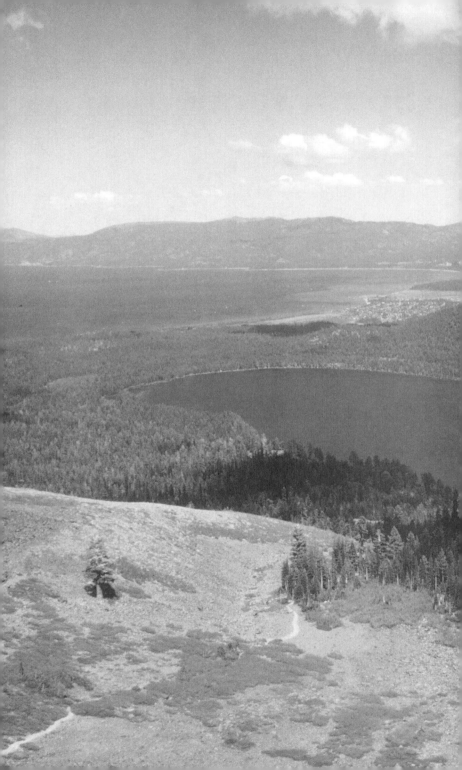

South Tahoe

The area around the south shore of Lake Tahoe contains some of the most picturesque and, consequently, most heavily used terrain around the lake. D. L. Bliss State Park and neighboring Emerald Bay State Park manage lakeshore tracts around Lake Tahoe that draw tourists and recreationists like a magnet to sandy beaches, picnic areas, campgrounds, and historical sites. Trails in these parks offer some of the best lakeshore views of Tahoe within the basin.

The 63,960-acre Desolation Wilderness, being blessed with an abundance of glacier-scoured lakes and granite peaks, is the most visited wilderness per square mile of any wilderness area in the entire country. The 105,165-acre Mokelumne Wilderness, south of Lake Tahoe, is a rugged landscape of volcanic peaks and lofty ridges that tower over deep canyons. The part of the wilderness that lies near Carson Pass is nearly as popular as Desolation.

Access to trailheads around the south shore of Lake Tahoe is straightforward via CA 89 and US 50, though summer traffic can be quite congested at times, especially in South Lake Tahoe. A mass transit system for Lake Tahoe has received considerable attention since President Bill Clinton's Lake Tahoe Summit in the 1990s, but more work is needed in order for the system to be effective. CA 88 services trailheads in and around the Mokelumne Wilderness.

Opposite and overleaf: *Fallen Leaf Lake (Trail 33)*

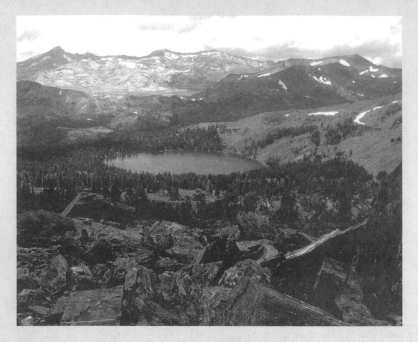

Gilmore Lake *and Pyramid Peak from Mount Tallac (Trail 31)*

Permits and Maps

The South Tahoe region is administered by a number of state and federal agencies. California State Parks oversees 6 miles of Lake Tahoe shoreline and 1,830 acres of surrounding lands in D. L. Bliss and Emerald Bay State Parks. Free brochures with sketch maps are available from the parks, or for online viewing at the state parks website, **parks.ca.gov.** Trails 24–26 occur within these parks. Both parks charge a nominal entry fee.

The Lake Tahoe Basin Management Unit and the Eldorado National Forest manage Trails 23 and 27–37, all of which enter Desolation Wilderness at some point. Available by self-registration at most trailheads, free day-use permits are required for all day hikes that enter the wilderness. In addition, parking at the Eagle Lake (Trail 27) and Pyramid Creek (Trail 37) trailheads is subject to a nominal fee.

Backpackers wishing to overnight within Desolation Wilderness have a rigorous set of hoops to jump through in order to secure a permit. Wilderness permits are required throughout the year, but an overnight quota is in effect from Memorial Day weekend through the end of September. Half the permits can be reserved ahead of time, beginning the third Thursday in April, either by phone at 877-444-6777 or online at **recreation.gov.** Within 14 days of departure, reserved permits can be printed online or picked up at ranger stations. The other half of the permits can also be picked up at participating ranger stations on a first-come, first-served basis.

In addition to the $6 reservation charge, fees are also collected for overnight use of Desolation Wilderness. Per-person costs for one night in the backcountry are $5 and $10 for 2 or more nights, up to 14 nights total. The cost of a single permit is not to exceed $100 per party. Children 12 and under are free. All fees are payable by credit card, check, or money order.

Trails 38–42 are within areas managed by the Eldorado National Forest. Currently, permits are not necessary for day hikes into the Mokelumne Wilderness, but overnight visits do require a free wilderness permit. Within the Carson Pass Management Area (CPMA), between Memorial Day and Labor Day weekends, a two-night limit is in effect for Round Top and Winnemucca Lakes (three-night limit for Fourth of July Lake), and camping is limited to designated sites. Permits for these campsites are available on a first-come, first-served basis from the Carson Pass Information Station. Campfires are not permitted within the CPMA or along the Blue Hole Trail, but are allowed below 8,000 feet within the rest of the wilderness.

The U.S. Forest Service produces excellent waterproof plastic topographic maps of both Desolation Wilderness and Mokelumne Wilderness at a scale of 2 inches equals 1 mile for $9 each. Maps are available from the Taylor Creek and Carson Pass visitor centers as well as from U.S. Forest Service headquarters and district ranger stations, or online from the National Forest Store at **nationalforeststore.com.** The USGS 7.5-minute quadrangles specific to this area are listed in Appendix 4.

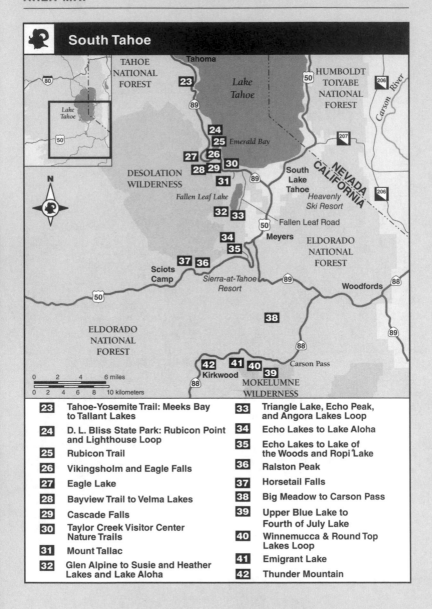

South Tahoe

TAHOE NATIONAL FOREST
Tahoma
Lake Tahoe
HUMBOLDT TOIYABE NATIONAL FOREST
Carson River
Lake Tahoe
Emerald Bay
NEVADA
CALIFORNIA
DESOLATION WILDERNESS
South Lake Tahoe
Heavenly Ski Resort
Fallen Leaf Lake
Fallen Leaf Road
Meyers
ELDORADO NATIONAL FOREST
Sciots Camp
Sierra-at-Tahoe Resort
Woodfords
ELDORADO NATIONAL FOREST
Carson Pass
Kirkwood
MOKELUMNE WILDERNESS

0   2   4   6 miles
0   2   4   6   8   10 kilometers

23	Tahoe-Yosemite Trail: Meeks Bay to Tallant Lakes
24	D. L. Bliss State Park: Rubicon Point and Lighthouse Loop
25	Rubicon Trail
26	Vikingsholm and Eagle Falls
27	Eagle Lake
28	Bayview Trail to Velma Lakes
29	Cascade Falls
30	Taylor Creek Visitor Center Nature Trails
31	Mount Tallac
32	Glen Alpine to Susie and Heather Lakes and Lake Aloha

33	Triangle Lake, Echo Peak, and Angora Lakes Loop
34	Echo Lakes to Lake Aloha
35	Echo Lakes to Lake of the Woods and Ropi Lake
36	Ralston Peak
37	Horsetail Falls
38	Big Meadow to Carson Pass
39	Upper Blue Lake to Fourth of July Lake
40	Winnemucca & Round Top Lakes Loop
41	Emigrant Lake
42	Thunder Mountain

TRAIL FEATURES TABLE

South Tahoe Trails

TRAIL	DIFFICULTY	LENGTH
23	4	16.0
24	1	2.0
25	2	5.0
26	2	2.5
27	2	2.0
28	4	10.5
29	1	1.5
30	1	up to 1.1
31	5	9.4
32	4	11.8
33	5	7.2
34	2–3	7.6–12.6
35	3–4	8.0–13.0
36	4	6.0
37	3	3.0
38	3	10.4
39	4	9.0
40	3	4.8
41	3	8.2
42	3	8.5

The table columns are: TRAIL, DIFFICULTY, LENGTH, TYPE, USES & ACCESS, TERRAIN, FLORA & FAUNA, EXPOSURE & OTHER (indicated by symbols).

Legend

USES & ACCESS
- Day Hiking
- Running
- Mountain Biking
- Horses
- Dogs Allowed
- Child-Friendly
- Wheelchair Access
- Permit

TYPE
- Loop
- Out-and-back
- Point-to-point

DIFFICULTY
- 1 2 3 4 5 +
- less more

TERRAIN
- Canyon
- Mountain
- Summit
- Stream
- Waterfall
- Lake/Shore

FLORA & FAUNA
- Autumn Colors
- Wildflowers
- Birds
- Wildlife

EXPOSURE
- Cool & Shady
- Great Views
- Photo Opportunity

OTHER
- Camping
- Secluded
- Historical Interest
- Geologic Interest
- Steep

South Tahoe

Eagle Lake 189

A short, popular hike along a tumbling stream to a beautiful subalpine lake, with an interpretive loop option, introduces sightseers to the characteristic beauty of Desolation Wilderness.

TRAIL 27

Hike, Run, Dogs
Allowed, Child Friendly
2.0 miles, Out-and-back
Difficulty: 1 **2** 3 4 5

Bayview Trail to Velma Lakes 194

Nestled in granite bowls, the Velma Lakes, along with Fontanillis and Dicks Lakes, are some of the most picturesque bodies of water within Desolation Wilderness, and give hikers the chance to experience some of the classic terrain for which the area is famous.

TRAIL 28

Hike, Run, Horses,
Dogs Allowed
10.5 miles, Loop
Difficulty: 1 2 3 **4** 5

Cascade Falls 199

A short hike to a picturesque, 200-foot waterfall will delight casual and serious hikers alike. Granite shelves above the falls offer fine picnic spots.

TRAIL 29

Hike, Run, Horses,
Dogs Allowed,
Child Friendly
1.5 miles, Out-and-back
Difficulty: **1** 2 3 4 5

Taylor Creek Visitor Center
Nature Trails 203

Four short and easy nature trails lead through a variety of habitats and picturesque environments, where visitors can sightsee, learn a bit about the history of the Tahoe area, watch for wildlife, or simply relax on a sandy beach.

TRAIL 30

Hike
Up to 1.1,
Out-and-back or Loop
Difficulty: **1** 2 3 4 5

Mount Tallac 208

One of Tahoe's most striking natural landmarks offers one of the area's most superb views. The efforts required for a stiff, nearly 5-mile climb are well rewarded at the summit, where expansive vistas await. Along the way are two pleasant lakes and plenty of scenery.

TRAIL 31

Hike, Run,
Dogs Allowed
9.4 miles, Out-and-back
Difficulty: 1 2 3 4 **5**

Horsetail Falls 239
Carrying icy meltwater from Desolation Valley, a thin
ribbon of feathery water plunges down the granite
headwall of Pyramid Creek's deep gorge, creating
one of the Tahoe area's most famous waterfall scenes.

Big Meadow to Carson Pass 245
Summer or fall, this trail takes visitors to some
grand scenery, including two expansive meadows
and two picturesque lakes. Colorful wildflowers tan-
talize the eyes in early season, while golden aspens
and meadow grasses provide visual treats later on.

**Upper Blue Lake to Fourth of
July Lake** 250
The back way into Fourth of July Lake offers
solitude and serenity, as well as some extraordinary
scenery in and around Summit City Canyon.

**Winnemucca and Round Top
Lakes Loop** 255
Recreationists are lured into the Mokelumne
Wilderness backcountry along a short loop trip
to two picturesque lakes backdropped by rugged
volcanic peaks. Fields of seasonal wildflowers and a
glimpse of a historic mine are bonuses.

Emigrant Lake 261
Stroll along the shore of Caples Lake's large reservoir enjoying the scenic views and then climb up
a stream valley to a glaciated cirque holding a gem
of a lake.

Thunder Mountain 265
The windy summit of Thunder Mountain provides
successful summiteers with expansive views of the
northern Sierra. The trail seems lightly used, with
most recreationists choosing the more heavily used
backcountry around Carson Pass.

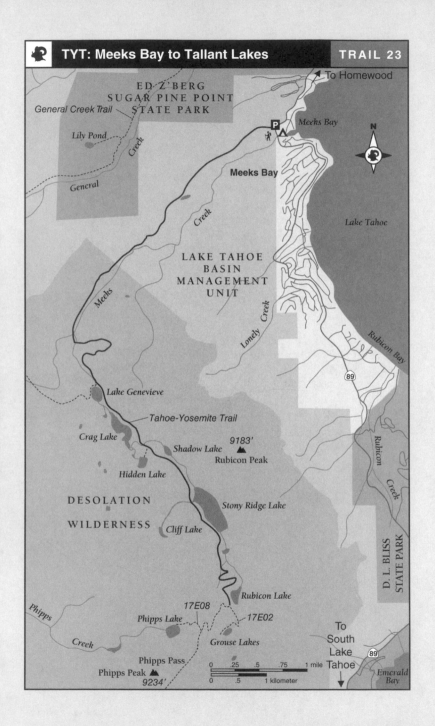

To Homewood

ED Z'BERG
SUGAR PINE POINT
STATE PARK

General Creek Trail

Lily Pond

Creek

General

Meeks Bay

Meeks Bay

Meeks Bay

N

Creek

Lake Tahoe

LAKE TAHOE
BASIN
MANAGEMENT
UNIT

Meeks

Lonely Creek

Rubicon Bay

89

Lake Genevieve

Tahoe-Yosemite Trail

Crag Lake

Shadow Lake

9183'

Rubicon Peak

Rubicon

Hidden Lake

DESOLATION

WILDERNESS

Stony Ridge Lake

Cliff Lake

Rubicon Creek

D. L. BLISS
STATE PARK

Rubicon Lake

Phipps

17E08

Phipps Lake

17E02

Creek

Grouse Lakes

To
South
Lake
Tahoe

89

Phipps Pass

Phipps Peak

9234'

Emerald
Bay

0   .25   .5   .75   1 mile

0   .5   1 kilometer

Tahoe–Yosemite Trail: Meeks Bay to Tallant Lakes

Along the north section of the famed Tahoe–Yosemite Trail (TYT), hikers follow Meeks Creek from its placid terminus at Meeks Bay upstream into Desolation Wilderness along a raucous course to its headwaters below Phipps Pass. The upper canyon boasts a string of seven picturesque lakes, precious jewels known locally as the Tallant Lakes, offering excellent opportunities for fishing, swimming, camping, or simply relaxing. Backpackers and equestrians with extra time will find plenty of connecting trails providing several options for lengthier journeys into the heart of the backcountry.

Best Time

Snow covers this section of the TYT until mid-July. Wildflowers are generally at their peak from late July–mid-August, but so are the mosquitoes. September offers mild weather, fewer people, and fewer mosquitoes.

Finding the Trail

Follow CA 89 to Meeks Bay and find the trailhead near a closed gate on the west side of the highway, 0.1 mile north of the entrance to the Meeks Bay Campground. The trailhead is approximately 16.5 miles north of the junction of US 50 and CA 89 in South Lake Tahoe, and 11 miles south of Tahoe City.

TRAIL USE
Hike, Run, Horses,
Dogs Allowed

LENGTH
16.0 miles, 8 hours

VERTICAL FEET
±2,200

DIFFICULTY
– 1 2 3 **4** 5 +

TRAIL TYPE
Out-and-back

SURFACE TYPE
Dirt

FEATURES
Canyon
Mountain
Stream
Lake
Wildflowers
Photo Opportunity
Camping

FACILITIES
None

Logistics

Overnight visitors must have a wilderness permit. The closest location to the trailhead to obtain one is the Taylor Creek Visitor Center.

Trail Description

▶1 Follow the gentle incline of an old dirt road across the north side of the broad, lush valley of Meeks Creek through a mixed forest of incense cedars, white firs, lodgepole pines, ponderosa pines, and sugar pines. After an easy 1.5 miles, the grade increases, as you forsake the old road at a well-marked junction and follow singletrack trail past verdant foliage near a seeping spring to the signed wilderness boundary, at 2.5 miles.

Beyond the wilderness boundary, the trail roughly parallels the creek, which is within earshot but mostly out of sight. Through alternating groves of conifers and pocket meadows you continue up the canyon to a log and timber bridge across the creek at 3.3 miles.

A moderate climb follows an arcing path around a red fir–forested side canyon filled with thimbleberry, fireweed, vine maple, and currant. Climbing

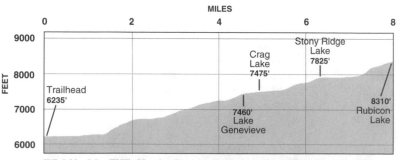

TRAIL 23   TYT: Meeks Bay to Tallant Lakes Elevation Profile

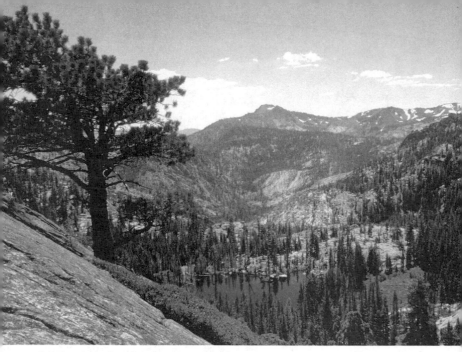

Granite slabs *along the Tahoe-Yosemite Trail*

out of this canyon, you circle around the nose of an open sub-ridge with a partial view of Lake Tahoe to rejoin Meeks Creek. A steady climb alongside the tumbling creek leads to a three-way junction marked by a 6- by 6-inch post, 4.6 miles from the trailhead. ▶2 The old Lake Genevieve Trail leading off to the right is a seldom-used lateral providing connections to the General Creek and Pacific Crest Trails. Just beyond the junction is Lake Genevieve, a greenish, shallow lake rimmed by pines. A number of fair campsites are spread around the far shoreline, but more appealing sites with better scenery are just a short distance up the trail at Crag Lake.

Follow the TYT around the east shore of Lake Genevieve and make a short, steady climb through western white pines, red firs, and Jeffrey pines to Crag Lake. ▶3 The lake has a splendid backdrop from the granitic slopes of 9,054-foot Crag Peak to the south. Overnighters should look for good campsites above the northeast shore.

 Camping

 Lake

Pass around the lengthy east shore of Crag Lake and ascend rocky trail to a boulder hop of Meeks Creek. Just past the creek, an unmarked use trail travels southwest to Hidden Lake, a shallow, irregularly shaped pond near the base of Crag Peak. A steeper climb through thick forest ascends some morainal ridges above the west shore of meadow-rimmed Shadow Lake, whose shallow waters are sprinkled with lily pads. A moderate climb follows the course of Meeks Creek, tumbling and plunging its way down the rocky canyon. At 6.3 miles you reach the north shore of Stony Ridge Lake, the largest of the Tallant Lakes. ►4 Except for the steep east shore, the lake is bordered by lodgepole pines. A number of excellent campsites will lure overnighters.

Camping Λ

Follow the TYT on a gentle grade around the west shore of Stony Ridge Lake, hopping over the outlet from isolated Cliff Lake along the way. Near the far end of the lake, a mildly rising ascent leads above the verdant meadow on the south shore and past a well-watered hillside carpeted with wildflowers. Eventually the trail resumes its climbing ways, switchbacking between the two upper tributaries of Meeks Creek, on the way to the last of the Tallant Lakes. At 8 miles from the trailhead, you reach the east shore of Rubicon Lake. ►5 Rubicon is perhaps the prettiest of the lakes, rimmed by mountain hemlocks and lodgepole pines, which shelter a number of excellent campsites.

🚶	MILESTONES	
►1	0.0	Start at trailhead
►2	4.6	Lake Genevieve junction
►3	4.9	Crag Lake
►4	6.3	Stony Ridge Lake
►5	8.0	Rubicon Lake

D. L. Bliss State Park: Rubicon Point and Lighthouse Loop

For good reasons, the Rubicon Trail is popular with hikers and tourists alike. Following above the lakeshore, travelers are treated to incredible lake views throughout the mile-long section of trail to Calawee Cove. By combining the Rubicon Trail with the Lighthouse Trail, you can follow a 2-mile loop, complete with Tahoe views and a bit of history at the old Rubicon Point Lighthouse.

Best Time

D. L. Bliss State Park is generally open from mid-May through the end of September.

Finding the Trail

Drive CA 89 to the entrance into D. L. Bliss State Park, approximately 11 miles north of the junction of US 50 and CA 89 in South Lake Tahoe and 16 miles south of Tahoe City. Proceed on paved road to the campground entrance station (fee required) and continue to the small parking lot on the left-hand shoulder, 1.1 miles from the highway. Both the Rubicon and Lighthouse Trails begin on the opposite side of the road from the parking area.

Trail Description

►1 Follow signs for the Rubicon Trail, to the right of the Lighthouse Trail, which will be your return route. Walk on wide and gently graded old roadbed through mostly fir forest, soon encountering the end of the road at a loop. ►2 Find the beginning of the

TRAIL USE
Hike, Child Friendly

LENGTH
2.0 miles, 1 hour

VERTICAL FEET
±550

DIFFICULTY
– **1** 2 3 4 5 +

TRAIL TYPE
Loop

SURFACE TYPE
Dirt

FEATURES
Shore
Great Views
Photo Opportunity

FACILITIES
Restrooms
Picnic Tables
Water
Phone
Visitor Center

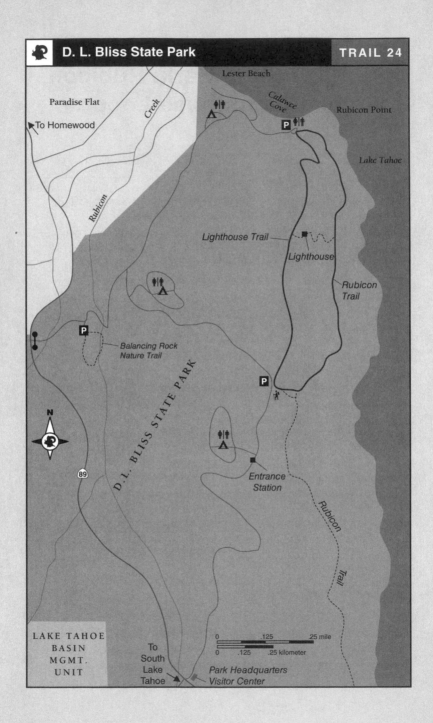

Paradise Flat

Creek

To Homewood

Lester Beach

Calawee Cove

Rubicon Point

Lake Tahoe

Rubicon

Lighthouse Trail

Lighthouse

Rubicon Trail

Balancing Rock Nature Trail

D. L. BLISS STATE PARK

N

89

Entrance Station

Rubicon Trail

LAKE TAHOE
BASIN
MGMT.
UNIT

To
South
Lake
Tahoe

Park Headquarters
Visitor Center

0   .125   .25 mile
0   .125   .25 kilometer

singletrack Rubicon Trail on the far side of the loop and turn left, obeying signage for Calawee Cove.

Proceed on well-maintained trail, where through the trees you can see Lake Tahoe and the peaks above the far shore. Soon scattered Jeffrey pines and firs allow better lake views, which improve even more where you reach open, shrub-covered slopes of chinquapin, manzanita, and tobacco brush. The excellent lake views continue until you come to a junction with a lateral on the left, which climbs the hillside to the lighthouse.

Past the lateral junction, you descend granite stairs to an unmarked path that travels a short distance to a vista point offering a superb Lake Tahoe view. Beyond the vista point, the main trail continues to the edge of a sheer cliff that you negotiate with the aid of a narrow boardwalk and chain fence. This area can be a logjam on busy summer weekends, as tourists queue up to wait their turn at the single-file passage. Once the crux of the route is safely negotiated, easier trail leads to the parking lot at Rubicon Point–Calawee Cove, 1 mile from the trailhead. ▶3

To continue the loop, follow the Lighthouse Trail from the parking lot on a mild to moderate climb, across a forested hillside to a switchback. As you climb away from the switchback, you may notice evidence of a previous fire. Eventually the grade eases where the trail nears the top of the ridge.

Rubicon Point Lighthouse's claim to fame is its elevation—the highest lighthouse in the world on a navigable body of water.

 Great Views

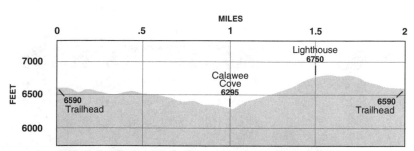

TRAIL 24 D. L. Bliss State Park: Rubicon Point & Lighthouse Loop Elevation Profile

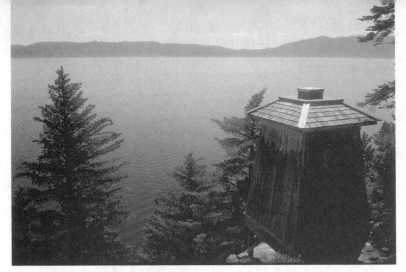

Rubicon Point *Lighthouse*

Proceed to a junction with a short path that leads down granite steps to the edge of the hillside and the restored Rubicon Point Lighthouse. ▶4 If you're familiar with seacoast lighthouses, you may be surprised at the diminutive stature of this lighthouse, which is about the size of a port-a-potty. However, what the structure lacks in appearance is more than made up for by the stunning view you have here of Lake Tahoe. Renovation and stabilization of the Rubicon Point Lighthouse was completed in 2001.

Away from the lighthouse junction, you continue to ascend for a brief time before the trail leaves the boulder-studded ridge and follows a moderate descent through mixed forest back to the trailhead. ▶5

		MILESTONES
▶1	0.0	Start at trailhead
▶2	0.1	Turn left (north) at junction with Rubicon Trail
▶3	1.0	Parking lot at Calawee Cove/beginning of Lighthouse Trail
▶4	1.5	Junction with trail to lighthouse
▶5	2.0	Return to trailhead

Rubicon Trail

If lakeside views across the sapphire-blue waters of Lake Tahoe are what you want, look no farther than the Rubicon Trail, which follows a 5-mile stretch of shoreline along Emerald Bay and the southwest shore of Tahoe, between Vikingsholm and Calawee Cove. Thanks to the beautiful scenery and the relatively easy route, the trail is popular with hikers and sightseers alike, especially on summer weekends. Plan on an early start to find a parking place and beat the crowds, though photographers will appreciate the lighting later in the day, when the sun is high or fading in the west.

Best Time

The Rubicon Trail stays close to the shoreline of Lake Tahoe, providing snow-free hiking mid-May–November. If you're hiking on a weekend between Memorial Day and Labor Day, make sure you arrive early, as the Vikingsholm parking lot fills up fast.

Finding the Trail

START: Drive CA 89 to the Vikingsholm parking lot above Emerald Bay on the west side of the highway, approximately 9 miles from the junction of US 50 and CA 89 in South Lake Tahoe and 18 miles south of Tahoe City. The parking lot is 0.25 mile north of the Eagle Falls parking lot.

END: Drive CA 89 to the entrance into D. L. Bliss State Park, approximately 11 miles north of the junction of US 50 and CA 89 in South Lake Tahoe and 16 miles south of Tahoe City. Proceed on paved road

TRAIL USE
Hike, Child Friendly
LENGTH
5.0 miles, 2.5 hours
VERTICAL FEET
+375/-700
DIFFICULTY
– 1 **2** 3 4 5 +
TRAIL TYPE
Point-to-point
SURFACE TYPE
Dirt

FEATURES
Shore
Great Views
Photo Opportunity

FACILITIES
Restrooms
Picnic Tables
Water
Phone
Campground
Visitor Center

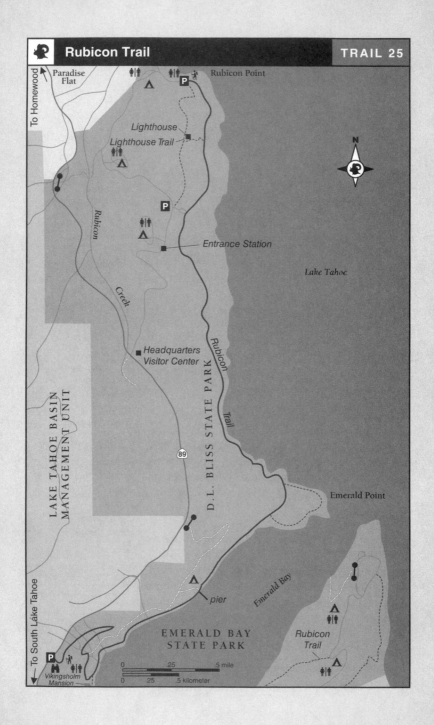

Rubicon Trail

TRAIL 25

Paradise Flat

To Homewood

Rubicon Point

Lighthouse

Lighthouse Trail

N

P

Entrance Station

Rubicon

Creek

Lake Tahoe

Headquarters Visitor Center

Rubicon Trail

LAKE TAHOE BASIN MANAGEMENT UNIT

D.L. BLISS STATE PARK

89

Emerald Point

pier

Emerald Bay

EMERALD BAY STATE PARK

Rubicon Trail

To South Lake Tahoe

P

Vikingsholm Mansion

0   .25   .5 mile
0   .25   .5 kilometer

past the campground entrance station (fee required) and past the small parking lot on the left-hand shoulder, 1.1 miles from the highway, where the Rubicon and Lighthouse Trails begin on the opposite side of the road. Continue on paved road another 0.5 mile to a stop sign at a T-junction and turn right, reaching the large parking lot at the end of the road, near Calawee Cove, 2.4 miles from CA 89.

Trail Description

▶1 Find a paved road at the northwest end of the parking lot and descend steeply along this road, which once provided residents and guests access to the Vikingsholm Mansion. Follow the road as it switchbacks 400 feet down the wall of the canyon above Emerald Bay, toward the mansion grounds at the bottom, where the Rubicon Trail begins near the lakeshore.

Head north from the beach area, passing outbuildings and picnic tables on the way to a number of bridges spanning small creeks and seeps that trickle down shady nooks filled with lush foliage. Proceed through mixed forest of incense cedars, Jeffrey pines, white firs, and sugar pines along the shoreline of Emerald Bay past Parson Rock, a hump of granite that provides shutterbugs with a superb

If you're not in a hurry, Emerald Point provides an excellent view of Emerald Bay and the surrounding terrain, including Maggies Peaks.

 Photo Opportunity

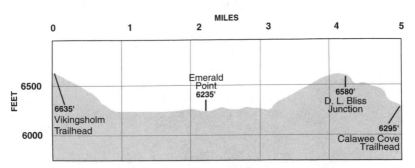

TRAIL 25   Rubicon Trail Elevation Profile

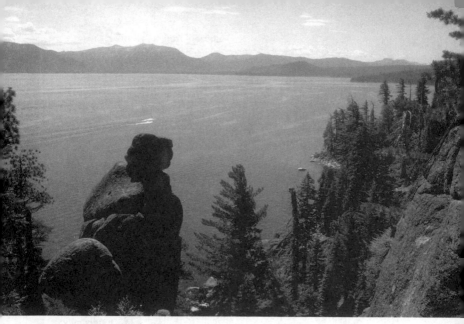

Rock outcrops *along the Rubicon Trail overlooking Lake Tahoe*

Tahoe view and swimmers with an excellent diving spot. Past the last of the bridges, you pass through Emerald Bay Boat-in Campground and continue along the trail past tall willows toward Emerald Point. At the start of this peninsula, 2.2 miles from the parking lot, a lightly used path veers right to follow the shoreline around Emerald Point, reconnecting with the Rubicon Trail 0.2 mile farther. ▶2

Beach 🏊

The Rubicon Trail climbs over a low moraine to the north junction with the Emerald Point Trail at a picturesque cove. ▶3 Nearby, a small stretch of sandy beach provides the last easily accessible piece of lakeshore until the end of the trail, at Calawee Cove. Climbing away from the cove, you reach a vista point at a pile of large boulders that provides a vantage point for a grand view of the lake. Follow a short, zigzagging climb and continue above the lakeshore before a short descent leads to a thimbleberry-lined stream spilling across the path. Farther on, after a pair of switchbacks, the trail veers away from the picturesque lake views to enter dense forest.

For the next mile, you make a steady climb through the trees to the trail's high point and then follow a short decline to a signed junction with the old road from D. L. Bliss State Park, 4.2 miles from the parking lot. ▶4 If time is of the essence, pickup could be arranged 0.1 mile away, at the Rubicon–Lighthouse Trailhead (see Trail 24), rather than at Calawee Cove.

From the junction, continue descending on well-maintained trail, enjoying filtered views through the trees of Lake Tahoe and the peaks above the far shore. Soon, scattered Jeffrey pines and firs allow better lake views, which improve even more where you reach open shrub-covered slopes of chinquapin, manzanita, and tobacco brush. The excellent lake views continue to a junction with a lateral on the left, which climbs the hillside to the Rubicon Point Lighthouse (see Trail 24).

 Great Views

Past the lateral to the lighthouse, you descend granite stairs to an unmarked path, which travels a short distance to a vista point offering a superb Lake Tahoe view. Beyond the vista point, the main trail continues to the edge of a sheer cliff that you negotiate with the aid of a narrow boardwalk and chain fence. This area can be a logjam on busy summer weekends, as tourists queue up to wait their turn at the single-file passage. Once the crux of the route is safely negotiated, easier trail leads to the parking lot near Rubicon Point at Calawee Cove. ▶5

MILESTONES

▶1	0.0	Start at Vikingsholm parking lot
▶2	2.2	South junction of Emerald Point Trail
▶3	2.3	North junction of Emerald Point Trail
▶4	4.2	Continue straight ahead at junction with trail to D. L. Bliss State Park
▶5	5.0	Reach Calawee Cove parking lot

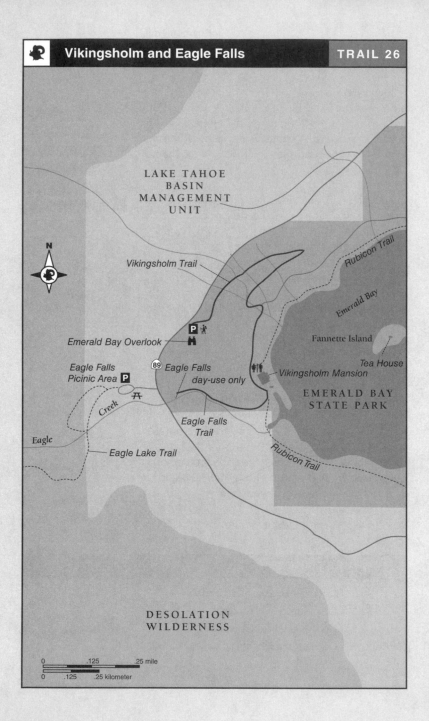

LAKE TAHOE
BASIN
MANAGEMENT
UNIT

N

Vikingsholm Trail

Rubicon Trail

Emerald Bay

Emerald Bay Overlook

Fannette Island

Tea House

Eagle Falls
Picinic Area

89 Eagle Falls
day-use only

Vikingsholm Mansion

EMERALD BAY
STATE PARK

Creek

Eagle Falls
Trail

Eagle

Eagle Lake Trail

Rubicon Trail

DESOLATION
WILDERNESS

0   .125   .25 mile
0   .125   .25 kilometer

Vikingsholm and Eagle Falls

Purchased by the state of California in 1953, designated a National Natural Landmark in 1969, and designated an underwater state park in 1994, Emerald Bay is Lake Tahoe's crown jewel. Along with a plethora of spectacular views, visitors to Emerald Bay State Park who come by boat or descend the 1.25-mile trail will find many diversions, including sandy beaches for sunbathing, excellent picnic spots, a vibrant waterfall, and the architectural wonder of Vikingsholm Mansion.

Best Time

The view of Lake Tahoe across Emerald Bay is spectacular any time of year, but snow-free trails beckon hikers and sightseers May–November. Eagle Falls provides the height of drama during peak flows when the creek is swollen with snowmelt from the mountains above, usually throughout the month of June. A tour of Vikingsholm Mansion (mid-June–September) is an absolute must for any visitor to Emerald Bay State Park. If your hike is planned for a weekend between Memorial Day and Labor Day, make sure you arrive early, as the Vikingsholm parking lot fills up quickly.

Finding the Trail

Drive CA 89 to the Vikingsholm parking lot above Emerald Bay on the west side of the highway, approximately 9 miles from the junction of US 50 and CA 89 in South Lake Tahoe and 18 miles south of Tahoe City. The parking lot is 0.25 mile north of the Eagle Falls parking lot.

TRAIL USE
Hike, Child Friendly,
Handicapped
Accessible

LENGTH
2.5 miles, 1.5 hours

VERTICAL FEET
±730

DIFFICULTY
– 1 **2** 3 4 5 +

TRAIL TYPE
Out-and-back

SURFACE TYPE
Paved, Dirt

FEATURES
Waterfall
Lake
Cool & Shady
Great Views
Photo Opportunity
Historical Interest

FACILITIES
Restrooms
Picnic Tables
Water
Phone
Visitor Center
Campground

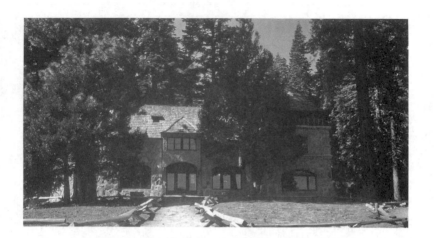

Vikingsholm

Mrs. Lora Josephine Knight, of Santa Barbara, secured the property around Emerald Bay, including Fannette Island, in 1928 for a price of $250,000. With her nephew by marriage, Lennart Palme, a Swedish-born architect, Mrs. Knight set out to design and build a structure that would be one of the finest examples of Scandinavian architecture in the western hemisphere. At great expense, the 38-room mansion was completed in September 1929 by employing 200 craftsmen using old-world techniques, such as hand-hewing large timbers, making intricate carvings, and fabricating hinges and latches. Following Mrs. Knight's wishes, not a single large tree was disturbed in the construction of her magnificent residence. Most of the construction materials came from the Tahoe Basin, including the granite stones in the foundation and walls. However, the furnishings inside Vikingsholm were either Scandinavian imports or meticulous reproductions of priceless treasures from Norwegian and Swedish museums. A handful of less spectacular outbuildings were also built, including the stone Tea House on Fannette Island. Servants would boat Mrs. Knight and her guests out to the island each summer day for afternoon tea. Mrs. Knight spent her summers at Vikingsholm, until her death in 1945. In 1953 the property was generously sold to the State of California for half its appraised value.

Logistics

You can camp on both shores of Emerald Bay, but the Vikingsholm area, including Eagle Falls, is only open 6 a.m.–9 p.m.

Trail Description

Before you head down to Vikingsholm, take in the view of Emerald Bay and Lake Tahoe from the nearby overlook. The vista is a Tahoe classic, and you will definitely want your camera if either the *Tahoe Queen* or M. S. *Dixie II* is visiting Emerald Bay. Tiny Fannette Island, near the west end of the bay, is the only island in Lake Tahoe.

▶1 After enjoying the view from the overlook, find a paved road at the northwest end of the parking lot and descend steeply along this road, which once provided residents and guests vehicular access to the Vikingsholm Mansion. Follow the road as it switchbacks 400 feet down the wall of the canyon above Emerald Bay toward the shady mansion grounds at the bottom. By obeying all signs for Vikingsholm, you'll reach the front of the magnificent mansion, 0.9 mile from the parking lot. ▶2 To tour the mansion, walk a short distance south to the visitor center and purchase a ticket ($5). Guided tours are conducted every half hour between 10 a.m. and 4 p.m.

Historical Interest

To visit Eagle Falls, find the start of the signed trail near the visitor center. ▶3 Head west on singletrack trail, paralleling lushly lined Eagle Creek through cool forest. Soon the grade increases and you climb shrub-covered slabs to a fenced viewing area near the base of the falls, 0.2 mile from the visitor center. ▶4

Waterfall

OPTIONS

Side Trips Along Emerald Bay

Hikers with extra energy can extend their trip by following the Rubicon Trail north from Vikingsholm to Calawee Cove along the shoreline of Emerald Bay and Lake Tahoe as described in Trail 25 (shuttle required). A shorter alternative follows the south shore of Emerald Bay through the campgrounds to Eagle Point and back.

MILESTONES

▶1   0.0   Start at Vikingsholm parking lot
▶2   0.9   Vikingsholm Mansion
▶3   1.0   Visitor center and Eagle Falls Trail
▶4   1.25   Eagle Falls

Eagle Lake

The short but steep 1-mile climb to Eagle Lake along the Eagle Lake Trail is one of Tahoe's most popular hikes, and for good reason. Where else can one visit such a picturesque lake tucked into an alpinelike granite cirque with such little effort? The U.S. Forest Service has recently built a short nature trail close to the trailhead, providing hikers and sightseers with an interesting and informative loop diversion.

TRAIL USE
Hike, Run, Dogs
Allowed, Child Friendly
LENGTH
2.0 miles, 1.5 hours
VERTICAL FEET
±450
DIFFICULTY
− 1 **2** 3 4 5 +
TRAIL TYPE
Out-and-back
SURFACE TYPE
Dirt

FEATURES
Canyon
Mountain
Stream
Waterfall
Lake
Photo Opportunity
Camping
Geologic Interest

FACILITIES
Restrooms
Picnic
Water

Best Time

Even though the backcountry beyond Eagle Lake remains snowbound until mid-July, the 1-mile trail to the lake is typically open by late June and usually remains snow-free until November. Parking at the Eagle Lake Trailhead is at a premium all summer long, so arrive early if you expect to snag a parking space, especially on weekends.

Finding the Trail

Follow CA 89 to Emerald Bay and locate the popular Eagle Falls Trailhead, on the east side of the highway approximately 9 miles to the north of the junction of US 50 and CA 89 and 19 miles south of Tahoe City. The trailhead is complete with picnic tables, barbecue pits, toilets, and running water. The U.S. Forest Service charges $5 per day for parking. Very limited free parking is available along the highway just outside of the trailhead parking area.

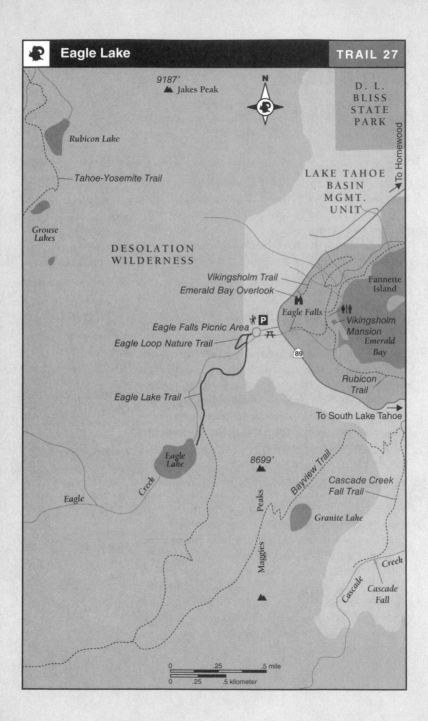

Eagle Lake

TRAIL 27

9187'
▲ Jakes Peak

N

D. L.
BLISS
STATE
PARK

Rubicon Lake

To Homewood

Tahoe-Yosemite Trail

LAKE TAHOE
BASIN
MGMT.
UNIT

Grouse
Lakes

DESOLATION
WILDERNESS

Vikingsholm Trail

Fannette
Island

Emerald Bay Overlook

Eagle Falls

Vikingsholm
Mansion

Eagle Falls Picnic Area

P

Emerald
Bay

Eagle Loop Nature Trail

89

Rubicon
Trail

Eagle Lake Trail

To South Lake Tahoe

Eagle
Lake

8699'
▲

Bayview Trail

Cascade Creek
Fall Trail

Eagle

Creek

Peaks

Granite Lake

Maggies

Creek

Cascade

Cascade
Fall

0   .25   .5 mile
0   .25   .5 kilometer

Logistics

Wilderness permits are required for both day hikes and overnight backpacks. Day hikers may self-register at the trailhead. Backpackers bound for the Velma Lakes and points beyond can obtain their permits from the Lake Tahoe Visitor Center, 5.5 miles south on CA 89.

Where else can one visit a picturesque lake in an alpinelike granite cirque with such little effort?

Trail Description

▶1 Climb away from the well-signed trailhead and follow wood-beam steps to a junction with the Eagle Loop Nature Trail, which is clearly marked by a 6- by 6-inch post. ▶2 Veer left at the junction and proceed through shrubs and scattered conifers, past a vertical cliff to the Eagle Creek Bridge, which is 0.2 mile from the trailhead. ▶3

From the bridge, follow granite steps across a field of blocky talus, soon crossing the signed Desolation Wilderness boundary. Past a patch of dense shrubs and lush trailside vegetation, you break out into the open across granite slabs, with grand views of Lake Tahoe and the towering cliffs rimming the canyon. Continue past scattered Jeffrey pines and junipers on a gentler grade, eventually encountering

 Geologic Interest

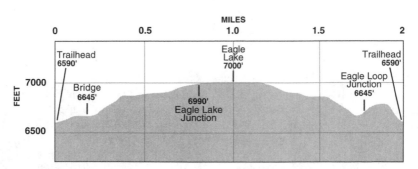

TRAIL 27   Eagle Lake Elevation Profile

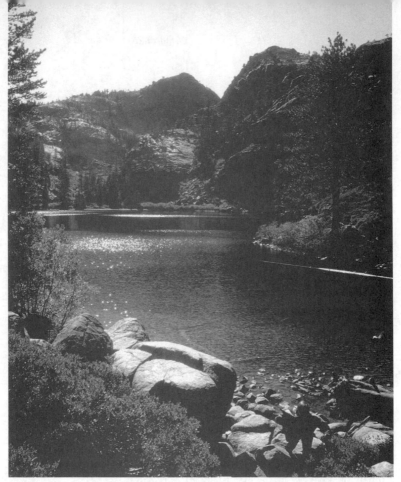

Eagle Lake

a denser forest of primarily lodgepole pines where the trail nears Eagle Creek. A short, stiff climb leads to a junction with the lateral to Eagle Lake, 0.8 mile from the trailhead. ►4

Take the lateral on the right and climb across shrubby slopes to the northwest shore of Eagle Lake. ►5 The scenic lake reposes serenely in an impressive granite cirque composed of steep cliffs. The shrub-covered slopes surrounding the lake, dotted with Jeffrey pines and white firs, offer limited access to the abrupt shoreline, providing a challenge for both swimmers interested in a chilly dip and anglers plying the waters for the resident trout.

You can vary the route of your return slightly by following the Eagle Loop Nature Trail. Immediately after crossing the Eagle Creek Bridge, ▶6 veer left at a junction with the Eagle Loop. ▶7 Just past an informational sign about the first sighting of Lake Tahoe by John C. Frémont and Charles Pruess, you reach another junction. The left-hand trail climbs granite steps and slabs to a viewpoint of Emerald Bay and Lake Tahoe, complete with benches and informational signs. The right-hand trail descends open slopes past more signs, to the lower junction with the Eagle Falls Trail. ▶8 From there, follow the main trail back to the trailhead.

MILESTONES

▶1	0.0	Start at trailhead; veer left (southwest) at Eagle Loop Nature Trail lower junction
▶2	0.2	Veer left (south-southeast) at Eagle Loop Nature Trail upper junction
▶3	0.2	Eagle Creek Bridge
▶4	0.8	Veer right (southwest) at Eagle Lake lateral
▶5	1.0	Eagle Lake
▶6	1.8	Return to Eagle Creek Bridge
▶7	1.8	Turn left (north-northwest) at Eagle Loop Nature Trail upper junction
▶8	2.0	Veer left (east) at Eagle Loop Nature Trail lower junction; return to trailhead

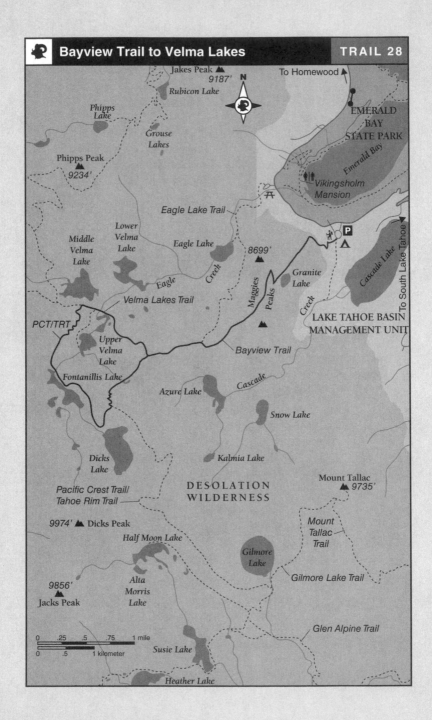

To Homewood

Jakes Peak
9187'

Rubicon Lake

N

Phipps
Lake

Grouse
Lakes

EMERALD
BAY
STATE PARK

Phipps Peak
9234'

Emerald Bay

Vikingsholm
Mansion

Eagle Lake Trail

Lower
Velma
Lake

Eagle Lake

8699'

Middle
Velma
Lake

Eagle   Creek

Granite
Lake

P

Cascade Lake

To South Lake Tahoe

Velma Lakes Trail

Maggies
Peaks

Creek

LAKE TAHOE BASIN
MANAGEMENT UNIT

PCT/TRT

Upper
Velma
Lake

Bayview Trail

Fontanillis Lake

Azure Lake

Cascade

Snow Lake

Kalmia Lake

Dicks
Lake

DESOLATION
WILDERNESS

Mount Tallac
9735'

Pacific Crest Trail/
Tahoe Rim Trail

9974' Dicks Peak

Mount
Tallac
Trail

Half Moon Lake

Gilmore
Lake

9856'

Jacks Peak

Alta
Morris
Lake

Gilmore Lake Trail

0   .25   .5   .75   1 mile

0   .5   1 kilometer

Glen Alpine Trail

Susie Lake

Heather Lake

Bayview Trail to Velma Lakes

This partial loop trip, consisting of 10.5 miles through the heart of the Desolation Wilderness, samples several cirque-bound lakes amid the characteristic granite terrain that makes the area so picturesque. Whether you're just out for the day or on an overnight backpack, the lakes provide great scenery, along with fine swimming and fishing.

Best Time

Desolation's backcountry is usually free of snow by mid-July. Wildflowers bloom from then until late August, when swimmers will find the water in the lakes the least chilly. The hiking season ends with the first major snowfall, which generally occurs in late October. On summer weekends, plan on arriving early to secure a parking space.

Finding the Trail

Drive CA 89 to Emerald Bay and locate the Bayview Trailhead on the south side of the highway, approximately 7.5 miles from the junction of US 50 and CA 89 and 19.5 miles south of Tahoe City.

Logistics

Wilderness permits are required for both day hikes and overnight backpacks. Day hikers may register themselves at the trailhead. Backpackers bound for the Velma Lakes and points beyond can obtain their permits from the Lake Tahoe Visitor Center, 4.5 miles south on CA 89.

TRAIL USE
Hike, Run, Horses,
Dogs Allowed

LENGTH
10.5 miles, 5 hours

VERTICAL FEET
±2,725

DIFFICULTY
− 1 2 3 **4** 5 +

TRAIL TYPE
Loop

SURFACE TYPE
Dirt

FEATURES
Canyon
Mountain
Stream
Lake
Wildflowers
Photo Opportunity
Camping

FACILITIES
Restrooms
Picnic Tables
Water

Trail Description

►1 Just past the trailhead, you reach a junction with the trail to Cascade Falls. Following a sign for Desolation Wilderness, turn right at the junction and make a stiff, switchbacking climb through mixed forest of primarily white fir with a chinquapin understory. Beyond the wilderness boundary you follow the crest of a ridge, where the forest parts enough to allow good views of Emerald Bay and Lake Tahoe. Leaving the ridge, the trail follows Granite Lake's alder-lined outlet and ascends through bracken ferns, thimbleberry, wildflowers, and a mixture of shrubs, including chinquapin, tobacco brush, and greenleaf and pinemat manzanita.

As you progress up the trail, lodgepole pines and western white pines join the forest on the way to serene Granite Lake, 1.0 mile from the trailhead. ►2

Near the far end of Granite Lake, the trail begins a switchbacking climb across the south-facing slope below the twin summits of Maggies Peaks. After a 0.75-mile climb, you bid farewell to the lake basin and follow mildly graded trail along the back side of South Maggies Peak to a gentle descent along the forested southwest ridge. At 2.7 miles from the trailhead, you reach a saddle and a signed three-way junction with the Eagle Lake Trail. ►3

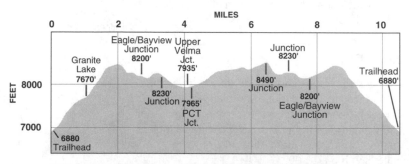

TRAIL 28   Bayview to Velma Lakes Elevation Profile

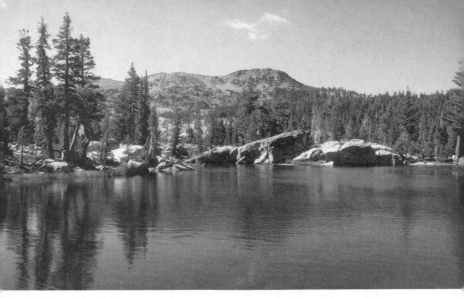

Upper *Velma Lake*

Veer left at the junction and follow sandy trail on a mildly undulating route through widely scattered mixed forest and around granite boulders and slabs. At 0.6 mile from the junction, you intersect the Velma Lakes Trail (17E34). ▶4

Bear right and follow the Velma Lakes Trail on a downhill course through acres of granite slabs, boulders, rocks, and widely scattered pines, which allow occasional glimpses of the unnamed pond directly north of Upper Velma Lake. Reaching the floor of the lakes basin, you walk along the north shore of the pond, ford the outlet, and come to a three-way junction marked with a 6- by 6-inch post, 4.1 miles from the trailhead. ▶5 Reach Upper Velma Lake via the trail to the left (south), which dead-ends after a half mile, near the inlet.

Continue straight ahead at the junction and make a short climb to intersect the Pacific Crest Trail (PCT), 4.25 miles from the trailhead. ▶6 A short walk northbound on the PCT leads to an unobstructed view of Middle Velma Lake.

Turn left at the junction and head south on the PCT on a moderate, winding climb above Upper

Velma Lake. Where the rate of ascent eases, Dicks Pass and Fontanillis Lake pop into view and then you make a short drop to the crossing of the lake's outlet. Cross Fontanillis Lake's multihued rock basin along the east shore of the lake, which lies in the shadow of towering Dicks Peak. Here, on the popular PCT, several campsites sheltered in groves of lodgepole pines and mountain hemlocks offer fine overnight accommodations for backpackers.

Camping

At the far end of the lake, a brief ascent across boulder-covered slopes leads to the top of a rise and the short lateral to Dicks Lake, where backpackers will find additional campsites. From the lateral, the PCT bends away from the cirque of Dicks Lake on a mild ascent to a junction with the Eagle Lake Trail, 6.4 miles from the trailhead. ▶7

A steep 0.3-mile descent from the PCT leads to milder trail, which traverses a pond-dotted basin. You reach the three-way junction of the Eagle Lake and Velma Lakes trails at 7.2 miles, closing the loop section. ▶8 From there, retrace your steps 0.6 mile to the Bayview–Eagle Lake junction ▶9 and then 2.7 miles to the Bayview Trailhead. ▶10

MILESTONES

▶1	0.0	Start at trailhead
▶2	1.0	Granite Lake
▶3	2.7	Turn left (west) at Eagle Lake Trail junction
▶4	3.3	Turn right (northwest) at Velma Lakes Trail junction
▶5	4.1	Go straight ahead (west) at junction with trail to Upper Velma Lake
▶6	4.25	Turn left (southwest) at Pacific Crest Trail junction
▶7	6.4	Turn left (north) at Eagle Lake Trail junction
▶8	7.2	Turn right (east) at Velma Lakes Trail junction
▶9	7.8	Turn right (southeast) at Eagle Lake–Bayview junction
▶10	10.5	Return to trailhead

Cascade Falls

A short hike leads to Cascade Falls, which during the height of snowmelt puts on a turbulent display of raucous watery splendor plummeting 200 feet down a granite cliff into Cascade Lake. Above the falls are several delightful picnic spots on granite slabs near swirling pools and tumbling cascades along aptly named Cascade Creek.

Best Time

Certainly, the best time to catch the falls at their peak is during the high-water period in June. The trail remains snow-free usually until late October.

Finding the Trail

Drive CA 89 to Emerald Bay and locate the Bayview Trailhead on the south side of the highway, approximately 7.5 miles from the junction of US 50 and CA 89, 19.5 miles south of Tahoe City.

Logistics

Wilderness permits are required for both day hikes and overnight backpacks in Desolation Wilderness. Fortunately, day hikers may register themselves at the trailhead. Maintained trail ends before the falls, requiring that trail users scramble over granite slabs and boulders to reach the best views. Adults should keep a close watch on young children at all times.

TRAIL USE
Hike, Run, Horses, Dogs Allowed, Child Friendly

LENGTH
1.5 miles, 2 hours

VERTICAL FEET
+75/-125

DIFFICULTY
- 1 2 3 4 5 +

TRAIL TYPE
Out-and-back

SURFACE TYPE
Dirt

FEATURES
Stream
Waterfall
Camping

FACILITIES
Restrooms
Picnic Tables
Campground
Water

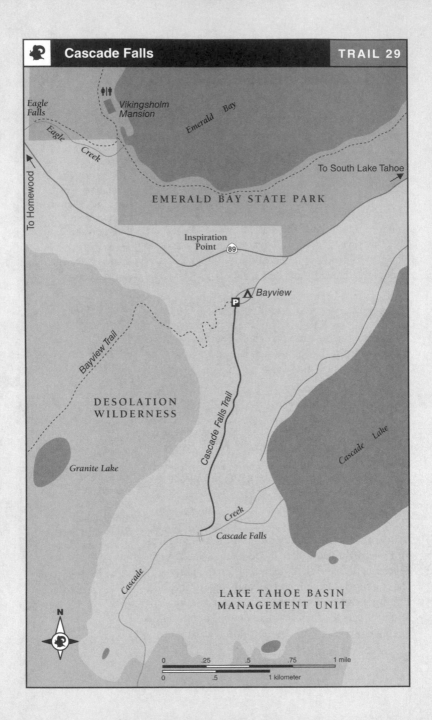

Cascade Falls   TRAIL 29

Eagle
Falls

Vikingsholm
Mansion

Emerald   Bay

To Homewood

EMERALD BAY STATE PARK

To South Lake Tahoe

Inspiration
Point   89

Bayview

P

Bayview Trail

DESOLATION
WILDERNESS

Cascade Falls Trail

Cascade   Lake

Granite Lake

Creek

Cascade Falls

Cascade

LAKE TAHOE BASIN
MANAGEMENT UNIT

N

0   .25   .5   .75   1 mile
0   .5   1 kilometer

Trail Description

►1 Just past the trailhead, you reach a junction with the trail to Granite and Velma Lakes. Following signed directions for Cascade Falls, turn left at the junction and climb over a low hill, then follow a gently graded path through a light covering of mixed forest and an understory of shrubs, including greenleaf manzanita, mountain chinquapin, and huckleberry oak. After a short climb over rock steps, picturesque Cascade Lake springs into view below, cradled in a glacier-scoured cirque basin. Unfortunately for recreationists, all but a slim portion of the eastern side of this lake is privately owned.

Follow the trail on a descending traverse across the west side of the basin toward the far end of the lake, and then start to climb over granite slabs and rocky sections of trail. Though maintained trail ends before the falls, use trails branch left toward the falls—simply follow the roar from the tumbling water. ►2 Exercise caution here, as loose rocks, slippery slabs, and overhangs could be potentially hazardous.

The tread of the use trails deteriorates a little past the slabs, but a series of cairns marks a faint

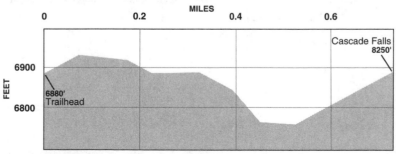

TRAIL 29 Cascade Falls Elevation Profile

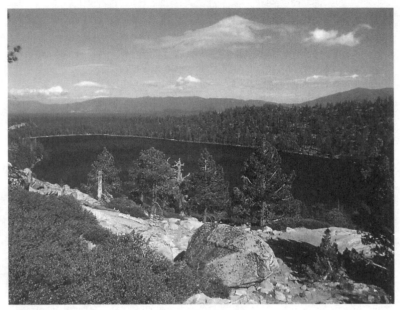

Cascade Lake *on the way to Cascade Falls*

path through dense foliage and then shortly loops through forest for those who wish to extend their journey beyond the falls.

🚶 MILESTONES

►1 0.0   Start at trailhead
►2 1.75 Cascade Falls viewpoint

Taylor Creek Visitor Center Nature Trails

Casual hikers, tourists, and sightseers flock to the Taylor Creek Visitor Center during the summer to enjoy a wide range of activities. A handful of short, gently graded nature trails provide opportunities to experience a number of diverse habitats and points of interest. The highlight for many is the Taylor Creek Stream Profile Chamber, where awestruck visitors have a belowground view of the creek and, in autumn, an opportunity to see Kokanee salmon during spawning season.

Best Time

Near lake level, the nature trails at Taylor Creek enjoy a long season, usually from late April to November. The highest visitation occurs between Fourth of July and Labor Day weekend. Early October is generally spawning season for the Kokanee salmon.

Finding the Trail

The Taylor Creek Visitor Center is located just off CA 89, 0.1 mile west of the intersection with Fallen Leaf Road. The well-signed turnoff to the visitor center is about 3.5 miles north of the Y-junction with US 50 in South Lake Tahoe.

Logistics

Summer weekends are quite busy at Taylor Creek. If you have the option, plan your visit on a weekday during the height of summer.

TRAIL USE
Hike, Child Friendly, Handicapped Accessible

LENGTH
Up to 1.1

VERTICAL FEET
Negligible

DIFFICULTY
– **1** 2 3 4 5 +

TRAIL TYPE
Out-and-back or Loop

SURFACE TYPE
Paved, Dirt

FEATURES
Stream
Shore
Lake
Wildflowers
Birds
Wildlife
Great Views
Photo Opportunity
Historical Interest

FACILITIES
Restrooms
Picnic Tables
Water
Visitor Center

203

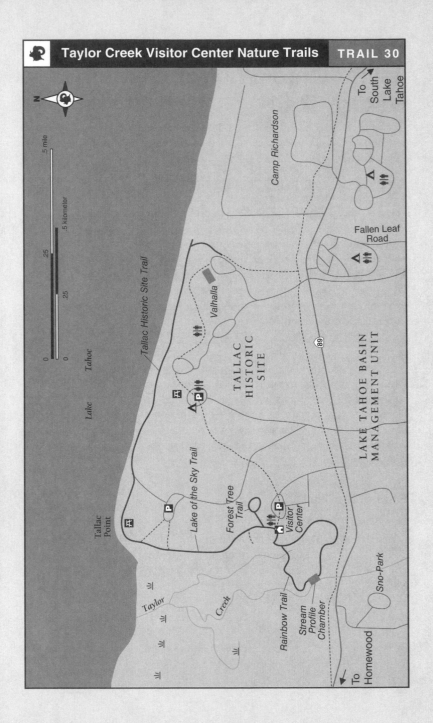

Trail Description

RAINBOW TRAIL: A paved, wheelchair-accessible path, augmented with interpretive signs, heads away from the visitor center past an aspen grove to a meadow carpeted with colorful wildflowers in early summer. Boardwalks guide you across boggy sections of the meadow while providing needed protection for the sensitive plant species that inhabit the wet soils. Park benches periodically placed around the loop and an overlook of the marsh, near where Taylor Creek spills into Lake Tahoe, offer peaceful spots to pause and ponder the majesty of the natural surroundings. After a quarter mile, the trail reaches the Stream Profile Chamber, where 12-foot-high floor-to-ceiling windows provide a below-water view of Taylor Creek. After a lingering visit to this unique perspective, follow the path on a loop back to the visitor center past more aspen groves and meadows.

 Wildflowers

FOREST TREE TRAIL: Though typically bypassed by most of the visitors to Taylor Creek, this extremely short nature trail is quite informative, offering visitors the opportunity to learn interesting facts about the Jeffrey pine ecosystem. Beginning on the north side of the visitor center, the loop trail passes several interpretive signs related to the Jeffrey pine and its relationship with other plants and animals in the forest.

LAKE OF THE SKY TRAIL: ▶1 Head south from the visitor center on paved trail to a junction with a paved path on the left that heads toward the amphitheater. Veer left and follow a gravel path through scattered Jeffrey pines and shrubs, then proceed alongside a three-pole log fence bordering a large meadow bisected by Taylor Creek. An elevated wood viewing deck provides an opportunity to scan the skies for a wide variety of birds, perhaps even

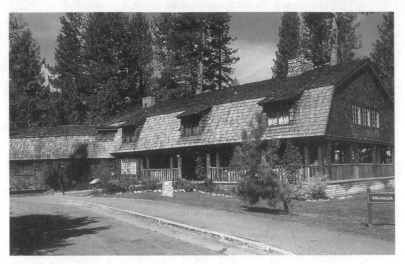

Valhalla Grand Hall *at the Tallac Historic Site*

a bald eagle in the off-season. Summer visitors can search the area for some of the 31 species of animals pictured on a nearby placard.

Away from the viewing deck, you pass more interpretive signs on the way to a four-way junction, where a lateral on the right heads east to a parking lot. Continue straight ahead at this junction and proceed toward Tallac Point, with Taylor Creek Marsh directly west of the trail and Baldwin Beach just beyond the marsh.

Reaching Tallac Point, ▶2 the trail bends east and follows the edge of the forest above a sandy beach along the shoreline of Lake Tahoe. Proceed through a scattered forest of firs, pines, and aspens to a Y-junction. Turn right here for a direct route back to the visitor center, or proceed straight ahead toward the Tallac Historic Site. Nearby a set of stairs provides access to the beach.

TALLAC HISTORIC SITE TRAIL: The Tallac Historic Site Trail can be accessed from either the Lake of the Sky Trail at Tallac Point as described above, or from the Kiva picnic area parking lot. Continuing west from the Lake of the Sky Trail, you pass an interpretive sign about the history of Lucky Baldwin's Tallac Resort. Nearby a concrete foundation is all that remains of the once elaborate structures that made up the resort. Heading away from this historical site, you reach the edge of the Kiva picnic area, complete with barbecue pits, picnic tables, and restrooms. A set of wood stairs nearby provides access to the sandy beach.

Beyond the picnic area, the trail continues eastward to a grape-stake fence near the boundary of the Baldwin Estate. On the other side of the fence, the path passes the estate's guest cabins and some larger structures, as interpretive signs provide insights into the area's history. Nowadays the Baldwin House is home to the Tallac Museum.

Past the Washoe Gardens and some park benches, you stroll through a gate into the Pope Estate, passing through an arboretum created in 1902 by the Lloyd Tevis family, the second owners of the property. The Pope Estate, the largest and oldest estate in the Tallac Historic Site, currently houses an interpretive center. At the far end of the property, the trail passes the boathouse, the boathouse theater, and the Valhalla pier as it meets the Tallac Bike Trail. The restored Valhalla Estate, currently used for community and private events, is just a short walk away. ▶3

𝕏	**MILESTONES**	
▶1	0.0	Start at Lake of the Sky Trailhead
▶2	0.4	Tallac Point
▶3	1.1	Valhalla

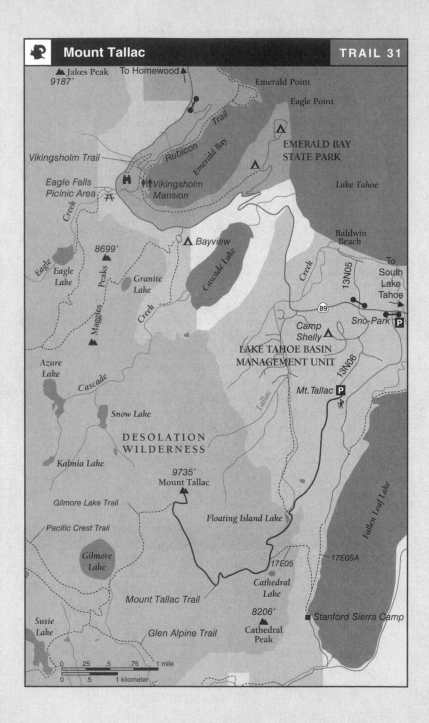

Jakes Peak
9187'

To Homewood

Emerald Point

Eagle Point

Rubicon Trail

Emerald Bay

Vikingsholm Trail

EMERALD BAY STATE PARK

Eagle Falls Picinic Area

Vikingsholm Mansion

Lake Tahoe

Creek

Eagle

Eagle Lake

8699'

Maggies Peaks

Granite Lake

Bayview

Cascade Lake

Baldwin Beach

Creek

13N05

To South Lake Tahoe

Creek

89

Sno-Park

Camp Shelly

LAKE TAHOE BASIN MANAGEMENT UNIT

Azure Lake

Cascade

13N06

Snow Lake

DESOLATION WILDERNESS

Tallac

Mt. Tallac

Kalmia Lake

9735'
Mount Tallac

Gilmore Lake Trail

Floating Island Lake

Pacific Crest Trail

Fallen Leaf Lake

Gilmore Lake

17E05

17E05A

Mount Tallac Trail

Cathedral Lake

Susie Lake

Glen Alpine Trail

8206'
Cathedral Peak

Stanford Sierra Camp

0   .25   .5   .75   1 mile
0   .5   1 kilometer

Mount Tallac

Mount Tallac is regarded by many as the quint-essential Tahoe peak. The dark, metamorphic hulk looms over the south end of the lake in dominant fashion, casting a long shadow over the surrounding terrain. *Tallac* is a Washoe Indian word meaning "great mountain," an appropriate moniker for this stately peak. Not only is the mountain imposing when viewed from various points around the basin, the vista from the summit is equally stunning. Prospective peak baggers don't need specialized mountaineering skills to reach the incredible view, as a maintained trail can be followed all the way to the top of the peak.

Best Time

At 9,735 feet, Mount Tallac holds onto its winter mantle well into midsummer—don't expect snow-free trails until after mid-July. At this altitude, high winds and winter weather usually signal an end to the hiking season on Mount Tallac during early to mid-October.

Finding the Trail

Drive CA 89 to Forest Route 13N06, which is opposite the road to the Lake Tahoe Visitor Center. Turn south on 13N06, obeying a sign reading TALLAC TRAILHEAD, and follow the paved road for 0.3 mile to an intersection. Turn left and proceed 0.2 mile to a junction with a road on the left to Camp Concord. Continue straight ahead at the junction, reaching the trailhead parking area at 1.0 mile from the highway.

TRAIL USE
Hike, Run,
Dogs Allowed
LENGTH
9.4 miles, 6 hours
VERTICAL FEET
±3,400
DIFFICULTY
– 1 2 3 4 **5** +
TRAIL TYPE
Out-and-back
SURFACE TYPE
Dirt

FEATURES
Canyon
Mountain
Summit
Stream
Lake
Wildflowers
Great Views
Photo Opportunity

FACILITIES
None

Logistics

Because part of the Mount Tallac Trail lies within Desolation Wilderness, you will need a permit for both day hikes and backpacks. Day hikers may self-register at the trailhead, but backpackers will need to get their permits from the Lake Tahoe Visitor Center.

Trail Description

▶1 From the trailhead, follow an old gravel road-bed on a mild climb through scattered Jeffrey pines and white firs. Beyond some backcountry signs the grade increases, the forest thickens, and on single-track trail you gain the crest of a moraine ridge. As you climb steadily along the ridge, Fallen Leaf Lake springs dramatically into view across a hillside carpeted with huckleberry oak and greenleaf manzanita. As fine as these views are, even better ones await farther up the trail. About 1.25 miles from the trailhead, the trail forsakes the ridge crest, drops briefly into a gully, and then on a steep ascent comes alongside the outlet from Floating Island Lake. Eventually, the grade eases and you reach the northeast shore of the serene, forest-rimmed lake, soon after crossing the Desolation Wilderness boundary, 1.7 miles from the trailhead. ▶2

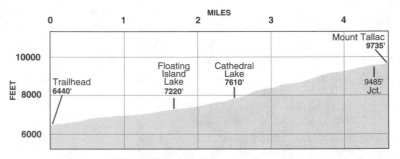

TRAIL 31 Mount Tallac Elevation Profile

Five-acre Floating Island Lake was named in the late 1800s for a 20-foot diameter, grass- and shrub-covered natural island that once sported thriving conifers. Since then several more grassy mats have sloughed off from the lakeshore and floated about the lake, though at the time of research, the surface was devoid of floating islands. The quiet lake is bordered by dense, mostly red fir forest.

Mild trail follows the shoreline past the lake and leads to a winding climb over rocky terrain and through thinning trees before it returns to dense forest and thick shrubs, alongside Floating Island Lake's inlet. Soon you break out of the trees and climb across an open slope carpeted with sagebrush, serviceberry, currant, and wildflowers, which allow fine views of Mount Tallac.

 Wildflowers

Back into the trees, the trail drops to a crossing of Cathedral Creek, lined with a luxuriant swath of vegetation, and then climbs to a junction with Trail 17E05. ►3 This trail provides a steep, exposed, 1-mile connection to Trail 17E05A, above the southwest shore of Fallen Leaf Lake. By following this trail to the north, you'll reach a tiny parking area in the Fallen Leaf Tract of summer homes. By heading south, you'll encounter Stanford Camp, the private university's extension campus, where there is absolutely no public parking and, therefore, no shortcut to Tallac's summit.

Continue climbing from the junction and soon reach Cathedral Lake, 2.5 miles from the trailhead. ►4 The diminutive lake sits in a steep rock basin surrounded by talus and sheltered by a few clumps of pines. Though reasonably attractive, the lake fails to inspire much reverential awe, having received its name from the nearby cliff on Tallac's southeast ridge.

Beyond Cathedral Lake the trail leaves the dense forest behind and attacks the hillside with a vengeance. On steep, rocky trail you climb across shrub-covered slopes with increasingly fine views of Lake Tahoe and the peaks rimming the southeast shore. A small brook adorned with wildflowers, including monkey flower, fireweed, larkspur, forget-me-not, and thimbleberry, provides the last reliable water for the remainder of the ascent. Long-legged switchbacks lead across slopes covered with tobacco brush, sagebrush, and bitterbrush, to the crest of Mount Tallac's southeast ridge.

Now heading northwest, you follow the ridge through wildflowers, shrubs, and groves of stunted conifers, including western white pines, mountain hemlocks, whitebark pines, and lodgepole pines.

Great Views

Improving views to the west of the Crystal Range peaks and the canyons of Desolation Wilderness are quite impressive. The steep ascent eventually leads to a marked junction at 4.4 miles with the trail to Gilmore Lake. ▶5

Veer to the right at the junction and continue the ascent over rocky slopes through diminishing

Summit

pines around the south side of Mount Tallac. As you regain the southeast ridge, Lake Tahoe springs back into view, and you follow the ridge the last 150 vertical feet to the summit. ▶6 At a mere 3.5 miles as the crow flies from the lakeshore, the top of Mount Tallac offers one of the Tahoe Basin's finest vistas.

🚶	MILESTONES	
▶1	0.0	Start at trailhead
▶2	1.7	Floating Island Lake
▶3	2.4	Proceed straight ahead at Trail 17E05 junction
▶4	2.5	Cathedral Lake
▶5	4.4	Veer right (east) at Gilmore Lake Trail junction
▶6	4.7	Summit of Mount Tallac

Glen Alpine to Susie and Heather Lakes and Lake Aloha

This trip provides a fine example of the classic Desolation Wilderness experience. An easy section of trail takes visitors to the historical setting of Glen Alpine Springs, before a moderate climb leads to three picturesque lakes in the shadow of Jacks Peak. John Muir's endorsement of the area reads, "The Glen Alpine Springs tourist resort seems to me one of the delightful places in all the famous Tahoe region. From no other valley, as far as I know, may excursions be made in a single day to so many peaks, wild gardens, glacier lakes, glacier meadows and alpine groves, cascades, etc." Don't anticipate huge doses of solitude, as this area is deservedly popular with hikers and backpackers alike.

Best Time

The short hike to Glen Alpine Springs can be done as early as the beginning of June, but the trail to the lakes is usually snow covered until mid-July. Patches of snow may remain over the trail in the upper cirque basins even longer.

Finding the Trail

Follow CA 89 to Fallen Leaf Road, approximately 3 miles northwest of the Y-junction with US 50 in South Lake Tahoe. Turn south and follow Fallen Leaf Road for 4.6 miles to the far end of Fallen Leaf Lake and a signed junction for Glen Alpine. Turn left at the junction and proceed on a very narrow paved road for 0.5 mile to the trailhead parking area, just past a bridge over Glen Alpine Creek.

TRAIL USE
Hike, Run, Horses,
Dogs Allowed

LENGTH
11.8 miles, 7 hours

VERTICAL FEET
±2,125

DIFFICULTY
– 1 2 3 **4** 5 +

TRAIL TYPE
Out-and-back

SURFACE TYPE
Dirt

FEATURES
Canyon
Mountain
Stream
Waterfall
Lake
Wildflowers
Great Views
Photo Opportunity
Camping

FACILITIES
Restrooms
Picnic Tables

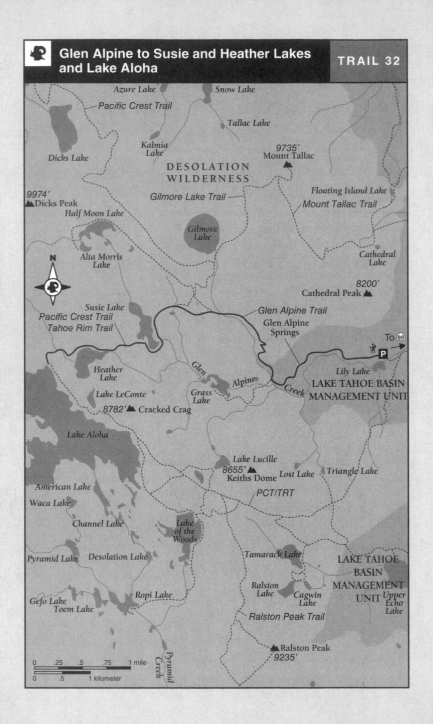

Azure Lake

Snow Lake

Pacific Crest Trail

Tallac Lake

Kalmia Lake

9735'
Mount Tallac ▲

Dicks Lake

DESOLATION WILDERNESS

Gilmore Lake Trail

Floating Island Lake

Mount Tallac Trail

9974'
▲Dicks Peak

Half Moon Lake

Gilmore Lake

Alta Morris Lake

Cathedral Lake

8200'
Cathedral Peak ▲

Susie Lake

Pacific Crest Trail
Tahoe Rim Trail

Glen Alpine Trail

Glen Alpine Springs

To 89

P

Lily Lake

Heather Lake

Glen

Alpine

Creek

LAKE TAHOE BASIN MANAGEMENT UNIT

Lake LeConte

Grass Lake

8782'▲ Cracked Crag

Lake Aloha

Lake Lucille

8655'▲
Keiths Dome

Lost Lake

Triangle Lake

American Lake

PCT/TRT

Waca Lake

Channel Lake

Lake of the Woods

Pyramid Lake

Desolation Lake

Tamarack Lake

LAKE TAHOE BASIN MANAGEMENT UNIT

Gefo Lake

Ropi Lake

Ralston Lake

Cagwin Lake

Upper Echo Lake

Toem Lake

Ralston Peak Trail

0   .25   .5   .75   1 mile
0   .5   1 kilometer

Pyramid Creek

▲Ralston Peak
9235'

Logistics

Backpackers will need a wilderness permit from the Lake Tahoe Visitor Center. Day hikers can register themselves at the trailhead.

Trail Description

►1 Begin hiking on a closed gravel road past private cabins and alongside lush riparian vegetation on the left, which obscures views of neighboring Lily Lake. The hillside to the right is covered with a mixed forest of junipers, Jeffrey pines, incense cedars, lodgepole pines, firs, and aspens. Continue along the road past Lily Lake to a scenic waterfall on Glen Alpine Creek and proceed to Glen Alpine Springs, 1.0 mile from the trailhead. ►2

 Waterfall

Dirt road continues beyond Glen Alpine Springs for a short distance, until singletrack trail climbs through mixed forest, followed by open, shrub-covered terrain with good views of the surrounding peaks and ridges. You enter the signed Desolation Wilderness and soon encounter a junction with the Grass Lake Trail, 1.6 miles from the trailhead. ►3

Turn right (north) and follow an extended, switchback climb over open granite slopes up the

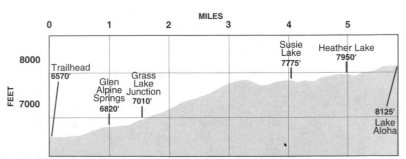

TRAIL 32 Glen Alpine to Susie & Heather Lakes & Lake Aloha Elevation Profile

Glen Alpine Springs

While searching for stray cattle in 1863, Nathan Gilmore dis-
covered the mineral springs that his wife, Amanda, would
name Glen Alpine Springs, after a verse in a romantic poem
by Sir Walter Scott. Gilmore built a wagon road to the springs
from Fallen Leaf Lake, bottled and sold the carbonated water,
and developed a first-class resort, which attracted several
noteworthy figures. A summer camp was established in 1878
and a post office in 1904, both of which were later relocated
to Fallen Leaf Lake. Several structures remain from the bygone
days, including the resort's social hall, a steel, redwood,
stone, and glass edifice designed by Bernard Maybeck, the
noted architect who also designed the San Francisco Palace
of Fine Arts. Nowadays, Glen Alpine Springs is under the
care of a nonprofit corporation, in conjunction with the U.S.
Forest Service, with a mission of preserving, restoring, and
interpreting the site's resources. The old social hall houses an
interpretive center, and guided tours and docents are available
on weekends from mid-June to mid-September. Glen Alpine
Springs also sponsors special events throughout the summer.
For more information, call 530-573-2405.

canyon of Gilmore Lake's outlet. Back under forest cover, you hop across an alder-lined rivulet,
continue climbing to a ford of the outlet, and soon
encounter a junction at 3.0 miles. ▶4

Veer left at the junction and follow Trail 17E32
toward Susie Lake. A short climb continues through
the trees and leads to a westward traverse past a
quartet of shallow ponds covered with lily pads.
Beyond the ponds the path descends to a junction
with the Pacific Crest Trail (PCT) near a wildflower-
covered meadow, 3.5 miles from the trailhead. ▶5

Wildflowers

Turn left and follow the PCT past two more
ponds and over a ridge to an overlook of rockbound
Susie Lake. A mild descent leads to a ford of the outlet near the southeast shore, a potentially difficult
crossing in early season. Named either for Nathan
Gilmore's oldest daughter or for the matriarch of
the Washoe Indian squaws in the mid-1800s, Susie

Lake is enchantingly cradled in a rocky bowl that characterizes the heart of Desolation Wilderness. ►6 The metamorphic hulk of Jacks Peak provides a fine backdrop to the long, irregularly shaped lake, which is bordered by clumps of heather.

Great Views

To continue to Heather Lake, follow the trail around the south shore of Susie Lake and make a steady climb toward the V-shaped notch of the outlet. Climb over the low, barren ridge to drop into Heather Lake's basin well above the shore, and continue toward the far end of the lake. ►7

Lake

A rocky trail climbs to a nice view of a waterfall and across Heather Lake's inlet. Continue the ascent past a placid tarn and to the crest of a ridge between the basins of Heather Lake and Lake Aloha. Here you have a marvelous view of the jagged Crystal Range, beyond the island-dotted surface of sizeable Lake Aloha. Dropping off the crest, you reach a junction with the Rubicon Trail at the northeast corner of Lake Aloha. ►8 The lake is most attractive in midsummer, before its level drops and it becomes a series of interconnected ponds.

🚶	**MILESTONES**	
►1	0.0	Start at trailhead
►2	1.0	Glen Alpine Springs
►3	1.6	Turn right (north) at Grass Lake Trail junction
►4	3.0	Veer left at junction
►5	3.5	Turn left at junction of Pacific Crest Trail
►6	4.1	Susie Lake
►7	5.0	Heather Lake
►8	5.9	Lake Aloha

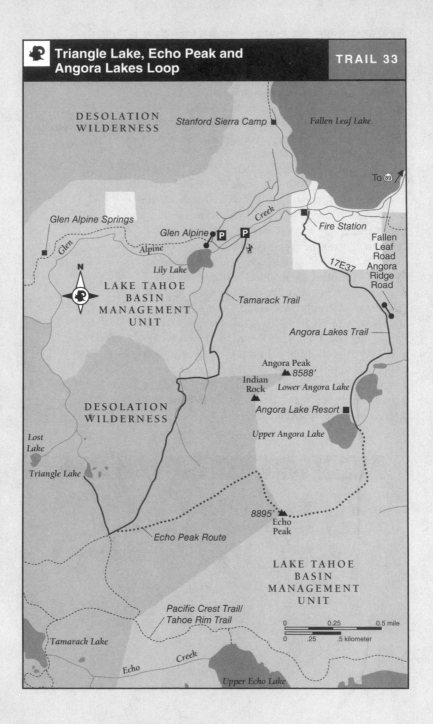

DESOLATION WILDERNESS

Stanford Sierra Camp

Fallen Leaf Lake

Creek

To 89

Glen Alpine Springs

Glen Alpine

P
P

Fire Station

Fallen Leaf Road

Glen

Alpine

Angora Ridge Road

17E37

Lily Lake

N

LAKE TAHOE BASIN MANAGEMENT UNIT

Tamarack Trail

Angora Lakes Trail

Angora Peak
▲ 8588'

Indian Rock
▲

Lower Angora Lake

DESOLATION WILDERNESS

Angora Lake Resort ■

Lost Lake

Upper Angora Lake

Triangle Lake

8895' ▲
Echo Peak

Echo Peak Route

LAKE TAHOE BASIN MANAGEMENT UNIT

Pacific Crest Trail/ Tahoe Rim Trail

0   0.25   0.5 mile
0   .25   .5 kilometer

Tamarack Lake

Echo   Creek

Upper Echo Lake

Triangle Lake, Echo Peak, and Angora Lakes Loop

Hikers searching for a more challenging adventure will find this loop trip right up their alley. Just locating the trailhead can be a daunting task for first-timers. From there, an unmaintained, primitive trail follows a stiff ascent up the canyon of the south fork of Glen Alpine Creek before gentler terrain leads to Triangle Lake and the summit of Echo Peak. The steep, off-trail descent from Echo Peak to Angora Lakes is the crux of the route, but a refreshing dip in the upper lake followed by a glass of fresh-squeezed lemonade at Angora Lakes Resort are worthy rewards. An easy hike along roads and trail completes the return to the trailhead. The views throughout the trip of Lake Tahoe and the surrounding terrain alone are worth the trip.

Best Time

Late July–mid-September provides the best conditions for the climb and descent of Echo Peak. Earlier in the season, some of the crossings of Glen Alpine Creek can be treacherous.

Finding the Trail

Finding the start of the trail may be the most difficult part of the trip. Follow CA 89 to Fallen Leaf Road, approximately 3 miles northwest of the Y-junction with US 50 in South Lake Tahoe. Turn south and follow Fallen Leaf Road for 4.6 miles, to the far end of Fallen Leaf Lake and a signed junction for Glen Alpine. Turn left at the junction and proceed on a very narrow paved road for one-third

TRAIL USE
Hike
LENGTH
7.2 miles, 5 hours
VERTICAL FEET
±2,750
DIFFICULTY
– 1 2 3 4 **5** +
TRAIL TYPE
Loop
SURFACE TYPE
Dirt

FEATURES
Canyon
Mountain
Summit
Lake
Wildflowers
Cool & Shady
Great Views
Photo Opportunity
Steep

FACILITIES
None

mile to the unidentified start of the Tamarack Trail.
Without a defined parking area or any signs marking the trailhead, a discernible path is almost impossible to spot from your car. The best plan may be to
first park your vehicle in one of the few spaces that
exist along the road, and then walk along the road
until you see the defined track of the trail on the
south side. If parking spots are not available along
the road, you will have to park your car at the Glen
Alpine Trailhead at the end of the road.

Trail Description

▶1 A short section of primitive trail leads away from
the road through open terrain to a 6- by 6-inch
post and a sign that would be much more helpful
if it were next to the road. After walking through
a small grove of Jeffrey pines, junipers, white firs,
and lodgepole pines, you emerge into an open area
of shrubs with nice views of the surrounding terrain, including Angora Peak and Indian Rock, high
above. Soon back in forest, you start a steep climb
Wildflowers on rocky tread through dense foliage. Aspen, thimbleberry, bracken fern, spirea, vine maple, alder,
willow, currant, and tobacco brush crowd the trail,
along with a colorful display of wildflowers, which

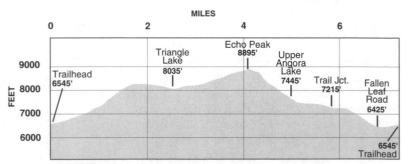

TRAIL 33 Triangle Lake, Echo Peak, & Angora Lakes Loop
Elevation Profile

includes columbine, leopard lily, lady slipper, and monk's hood. Eventually the junglelike vegetation is left behind, as the stiff ascent continues across shrub-covered and boulder-dotted slopes with scattered conifers that allow improving views of Lake Tahoe, Fallen Leaf Lake, and the nearby topography. As you continue the climb up the canyon, you make several crossings of the thin, lushly lined stream, as mountain hemlocks and western white pines join the scattered forest.

Eventually the stiff climb abates as you reach the top of the canyon and follow gently graded trail through scattered timber and drier vegetation of grasses, sedges, sagebrush, and assorted wildflowers, mainly lupine. At 2.2 miles, you pass an unmarked trail on the left, angling sharply away from the main trail, which will soon be your route to Echo Peak. ▶2 Continue on the main trail about 100 yards farther, to the signed, four-way junction with a lateral to Triangle Lake on the right. ▶3

To visit Triangle Lake, head north on a mild descent through mixed forest and past small, flower-filled meadows. After a quarter mile the descent becomes steeper, eventually leading across a boggy meadow to the south shore of secluded Triangle Lake. ▶4 The serene lake is sandwiched between low rock hummocks and surrounded by scattered conifers.

Retrace your steps 0.3 mile to the four-way junction ▶3 and then 100 yards to the unmarked junction of the route to Echo Peak. ▶2 Head northeast (right) on a mild to moderate climb through a mixed forest of lodgepole pines, western white pines, mountain hemlocks, whitebark pines, and white firs. After 0.8 mile you emerge from the forest and reach the low point of a ridge crest between Indian Rock and Echo Peak. From the brink of the ridge, you gaze straight down a nearly vertical cliff to shimmering Angora Lakes, 1,300 feet below. Turn right and follow a

 Summit

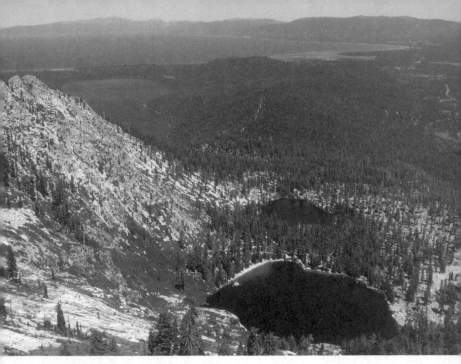

Looking down *at Angora Lakes*

Great Views

Steep

ducked route along the crest, toward the granite blocks that form Echo Peak's summit, where you'll enjoy a marvelous 360-degree view. ►5 Some of the more notable Tahoe landmarks visible from the summit are Mount Tallac, the Crystal Range, and the peaks near Carson Pass.

After reveling in the summit view, follow a well-defined path along the southeast ridge of Echo Peak for a short distance and then descend steeply down the northeast ridge toward the east side of Upper Angora Lake. Several descent routes seem to come and go, but the general route is easy to determine. Around 7,775 feet, you reach a small flat southeast of the lake, where your knees will enjoy the temporary reprieve from the steep descent. Away from the flat, descend a steep hillside, cross a talus field, and reach the east shore of the upper lake. ►6

On a typical summer day you're apt to have plenty of company here, as the family-run Angora Lakes Resort manages a large sandy beach, boat rentals, a snack shop, and eight housekeeping cabins, all of which make Upper Angora Lake a popular destination for swimmers, sunbathers, boaters, and sightseers. Both lakes are stocked with trout, attracting many anglers as well. High, granite ledges above the south shore lure adventurous divers, but exercise caution—there have been a number of fatal accidents involving divers at the upper lake. On a brighter note, the fresh-squeezed lemonade from the snack shop is reportedly excellent.

From the upper lake, follow the wide road above the west shore of Lower Angora Lake, which, despite the presence of several summer cabins along the far shore, is much more serene than the upper lake. Remain on the road for a quarter mile past the lower lake to the parking lot and continue to the far end, where the trail to Fallen Leaf Lake begins. ►7 Though the trail is unmarked at the start, a 6- by 6-inch signpost a short distance down the path provides assurance that you're on the right route.

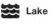 Lake

Leaving the hustle and bustle of Angora Lakes, a slightly rising trail amid white firs and lodgepole pines leads to a short and steep climb to the crest of a ridge, where through the trees you have filtered views of Fallen Leaf Lake and Mount Tallac. A long angling descent incorporating a few switchbacks cuts across the hillside above the south shore of Fallen Leaf Lake. Farther down the slope, you encounter pockets of dense, head-high foliage alternating with open areas that provide excellent views across the lake. A final series of short switchbacks takes you back into the trees and down to Fallen Leaf Road near the fire station and a chapel. ►8 From there walk the road to Glen Alpine 0.3 mile, back to the start of the Tamarack Trail. ►9

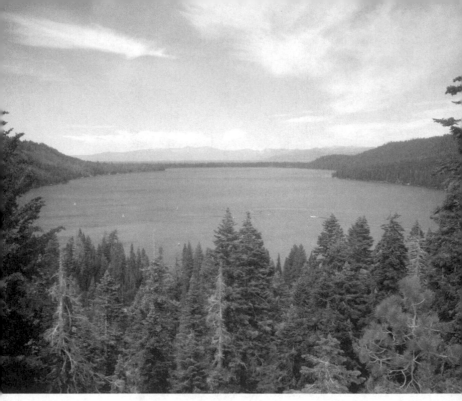

Fallen Leaf Lake

🚶	**MILESTONES**	
▶1	0.0	Start at trailhead
▶2	2.2	Continue straight ahead (southwest) at use trail to Echo Peak
▶3	2.25	Turn right (north) at Triangle Lake junction
▶4	2.6	Triangle Lake
▶3	3.05	Backtrack to Triangle Lake junction
▶2	3.0	Backtrack to start of use trail to Echo Peak
▶5	4.1	Summit of Echo Peak
▶6	5.0	Upper Angora Lake
▶7	5.7	Start of trail to Fallen Leaf Lake
▶8	6.7	Fallen Leaf Road
▶9	7.2	Return to trailhead

Echo Lakes to Lake Aloha

This section of the famed Pacific Crest Trail (PCT) is perhaps the most popular route into the heart of Desolation Wilderness. The relatively high elevation start coupled with the ability to shave off 2.5 miles of hiking by taking the water taxi across the lakes make this a highly desirable entry point for backcountry enthusiasts. With a bounty of scenic lakes and plenty of dramatic mountain scenery so easily accessible, the area's popularity is no mystery. While backpackers contend for a limited number of wilderness permits, hikers are free to roam the backcountry within a day's journey at will—just don't expect to be alone.

Best Time

Hikers will typically find snow-free trails mid-July–mid-October. The water taxi runs from the Fourth of July to Labor Day weekend, with limited service after that, usually through September.

Finding the Trail

From US 50, about 1.25 miles west of Echo Summit and 1.8 miles east of Sierra-at-Tahoe ski resort, following a sign for Berkeley Camp and Echo Lakes, turn east onto Johnson Pass Road and travel 0.5 mile and then turn left at Echo Lakes Road. Continue up

TRAIL USE
Hike, Run, Horses,
Dogs Allowed,
Child Friendly
LENGTH*
VERTICAL FEET*
DIFFICULTY*
*See table below
TRAIL TYPE
Out-and-back
SURFACE TYPE
Dirt

FEATURES
Mountain
Lake
Wildflowers
Photo Opportunity
Camping

FACILITIES
Restrooms

🚶 DESTINATIONS	LENGTH	VERTICAL FEET	DIFFICULTY
WITH WATER TAXI	7.6 miles, 4 hours	+3,425	– 1 **2** 3 4 5 +
WITHOUT WATER TAXI	12.6 miles, 7 hours	+1,725	– 1 2 **3** 4 5 +

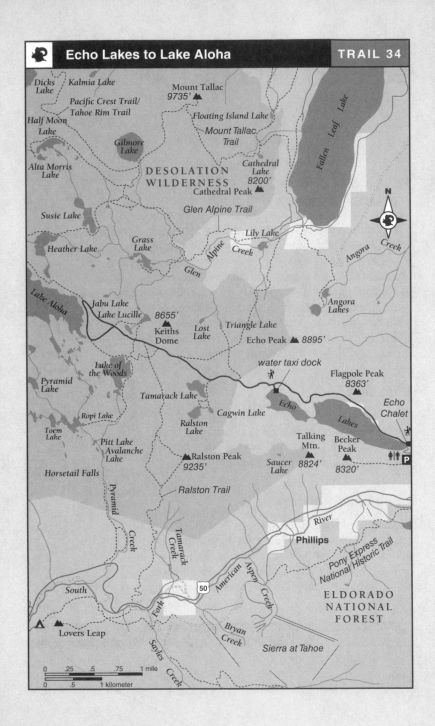

Dicks Lake

Kalmia Lake

Pacific Crest Trail/ Tahoe Rim Trail

Mount Tallac
9735'

Floating Island Lake

Half Moon Lake

Mount Tallac Trail

Fallen Leaf Lake

Gilmore Lake

Alta Morris Lake

DESOLATION WILDERNESS

Cathedral Lake
8200'

Cathedral Peak

Glen Alpine Trail

Susie Lake

Lily Lake

Grass Lake

Alpine Creek

Heather Lake

Angora Creek

Glen

Lake Aloha

Jabu Lake
Lake Lucille

8655'

Keiths Dome

Lost Lake

Triangle Lake

Echo Peak 8895'

Angora Lakes

water taxi dock

Flagpole Peak
8363'

Lake of the Woods

Pyramid Lake

Echo

Echo Chalet

Tamarack Lake

Cagwin Lake

Lakes

Ropi Lake

Ralston Lake

Talking Mtn.
8824'

Becker Peak
8320'

Toem Lake

Pitt Lake
Avalanche Lake

Ralston Peak
9235'

Saucer Lake

P

Horsetail Falls

Pyramid Creek

Ralston Trail

River

Tamarack Creek

Phillips

Pony Express National Historic Trail

South

50

American

Aspen Creek

ELDORADO NATIONAL FOREST

Fork

Lovers Leap

Bryan Creek

Sierra at Tahoe

Sayles Creek

0   .25   .5   .75   1 mile
0   .5   1 kilometer

this road for 0.9 mile to the large trailhead parking area above the south shore of Lower Echo Lake.

Logistics

The Echo Lake Chalet offers water taxi service from the resort's dock at the south end of Lower Echo Lake to the public dock at the far end of Upper Echo Lake, reducing the hiking distance by 2.5 miles. The normal season runs from the Fourth of July through Labor Day weekend, though service usually extends through September, depending on weather conditions and lake levels. At the time of research, the fee was $12 per person, one-way, with a $36 per boatload minimum (dogs are $5 each). A direct phone line from the upper dock to the chalet can be used to arrange for pickup. When the channel to the upper lake is no longer navigable, usually by mid-September, passengers are dropped at the end of the lower lake for a reduced fee with a four-person minimum. Call 530-659-7207 (8 a.m.–6 p.m., summer only) for more information, or visit the website at **echochalet.com.**

Trail Description

Without water taxi service, you'll have to walk the extra 2.5 miles around the north shore of Echo

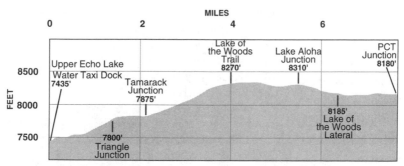

TRAIL 34 Echo Lakes to Lake Aloha Elevation Profile

Lakes and add that distance to the following mileages. ►1 From the water taxi pier, climb to the junction with the Pacific Crest Trail (PCT). ►2 Turn left (west) and proceed on rocky tread across open slopes on a westbound course, away from the lakes. Near the Desolation Wilderness boundary, 0.7 mile from the pier, you meet a junction with a lightly used trail to Triangle Lake. ►3 Another 0.4 mile of hiking leads to a junction with a lateral to Tamarack, Ralston, and Cagwin Lakes. ►4 These three picturesque lakes are worth a visit if you have the extra time and energy.

Lake 〰〰

Beyond the junction, the PCT follows a moderate climb to a diminutive rivulet coursing through a ravine and then continues the ascent via a pair of switchbacks to an open bench and a junction with the Tamarack Trail, 1.1 miles from the pier. ►5

Gently ascending trail brings you along the northern fringe of the broad expanse of grass-covered Haypress Meadows, where early- to mid-summer wildflowers put on a fine floral display. Near the far end of the meadows, at 2.0 miles, is the junction with Trail 17E40 to Lake of the Woods (see Trail 35). ►6

Wildflowers ✿

After a quarter-mile stroll from the Lake of the Woods junction, you pass the lightly used Ralston Peak Trail near the high point of the journey and continue toward Lake Aloha. Reach another junction (after a mere 0.1 mile) with the east end of Trail 17E09 to Lake Margery and Lake Lucille on the right. ►7 The 0.7-mile trail makes a fine diversion for a slight variation on the return trip. Proceed along the gently graded PCT to the Lake Aloha Trail, at 2.75 miles from the pier. ►8

With a bounty of scenic lakes and plenty of dramatic mountain scenery so easily accessible, the area's popularity is no mystery.

Leave the PCT and turn left onto the Lake Aloha Trail heading southwest toward the sprawling lake. After 0.4 mile, pass a lateral heading southeast to Lake of the Woods. ►9 A short distance later encounter an unmarked path on the left that leads

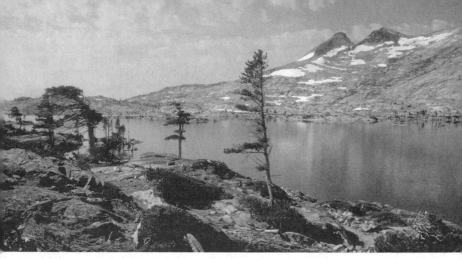

Lake Aloha

to Lake Aloha's dam, where swimming can be quite pleasant when the water level is accommodating. Continuing north on the main trail takes you along the east shore of Lake Aloha to a reunion with the PCT at 3.8 miles. ►10 Turn right (southeast) and follow the PCT back to the pier at Upper Echo Lake and call for the water taxi. ►11 Without taxi service, you'll have to hike the 2.5 miles back to the parking lot at Lower Echo Lake.

🚶	MILESTONES		
►1	0.0	2.5	Start at Upper Echo Lake pier
►2	0.1	2.6	Turn left (west) at PCT junction
►3	0.7	3.2	Continue straight ahead at Triangle Lake junction
►4	1.1	3.6	Continue straight ahead at Tamarack Lake junction
►5	2.0	4.5	Continue straight ahead at Lake of the Woods junction
►6	2.25	4.75	Continue straight ahead at Ralston Peak junction
►7	2.35	4.85	Continue straight ahead at Lake Margery junction
►8	2.75	5.25	Turn left (southwest) onto Lake Aloha Trail
►9	3.2	5.7	Veer right at lateral to Lake of the Woods
►10	3.8	6.3	Turn right (southeast) at PCT junction
►11	7.6	10.1	Return to Upper Echo Lake pier

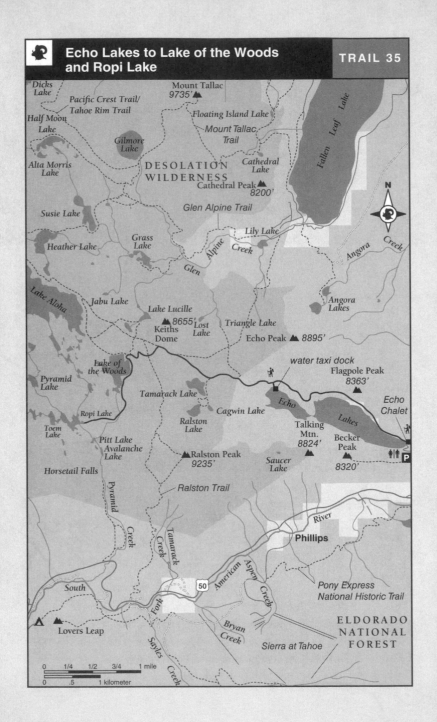

Dicks Lake

Pacific Crest Trail/ Tahoe Rim Trail

Half Moon Lake

Mount Tallac 9735'

Floating Island Lake

Mount Tallac Trail

Gilmore Lake

Fallen Leaf Lake

Alta Morris Lake

DESOLATION WILDERNESS

Cathedral Lake

Cathedral Peak 8200'

N

Susie Lake

Glen Alpine Trail

Lily Lake

Heather Lake

Grass Lake

Alpine Creek

Angora Creek

Glen

Lake Aloha

Jabu Lake

Lake Lucille

Triangle Lake

Angora Lakes

8655'
Keiths Dome

Lost Lake

Echo Peak 8895'

Pyramid Lake

Lake of the Woods

Tamarack Lake

Cagwin Lake

water taxi dock

Flagpole Peak 8363'

Echo Chalet

Ropi Lake

Ralston Lake

Echo

Lakes

Toem Lake

Pitt Lake Avalanche Lake

Ralston Peak 9235'

Talking Mtn. 8824'

Becker Peak 8320'

Horsetail Falls

Saucer Lake

Ralston Trail

Pyramid Creek

Tamarack Creek

River

Phillips

South

50

American

Aspen Creek

Pony Express National Historic Trail

Lovers Leap

Fork

Sayles Creek

Bryan Creek

Sierra at Tahoe

ELDORADO NATIONAL FOREST

0   1/4   1/2   3/4   1 mile
0   .5   1 kilometer

Echo Lakes to Lake of the Woods and Ropi Lake

Lake of the Woods, with numerous coves, islands, and campsites, is a popular destination accessible by maintained trail. The rest of Desolation Valley beyond Lake of the Woods is one of the most picturesque corners of Desolation Wilderness. Beneath the rugged east face of majestic Pyramid Peak, the granite, glacier-scoured basin holds a plethora of lakes and ponds, most of which are not accessible by developed and maintained trail. Hikers and backpackers with rudimentary cross-country skills have a fantastic playground for exploration of the nooks and crannies of this alpinelike basin.

Best Time

Hikers will typically find snow-free trails mid-July–mid-October. The water taxi runs from the Fourth of July to Labor Day weekend, with limited service after that, usually through September.

Finding the Trail

From US 50, about 1.25 miles west of Echo Summit and 1.8 miles east of the Sierra-at-Tahoe ski resort, following a sign for Berkeley Camp and Echo Lakes, turn east onto Johnson Pass Road and travel 0.5 mile and then turn left at Echo Lakes Road. Continue up

TRAIL USE
Hike, Run, Bike, Dogs
Allowed, Child Friendly

LENGTH*

VERTICAL FEET*

DIFFICULTY*
*See table below

TRAIL TYPE
Out-and-back

SURFACE TYPE
Dirt

FEATURES
Canyon
Mountain
Summit
Stream
Waterfall
Shore
Autumn Colors
Wildflowers
Birds
Wildlife
Cool & Shady
Camping

FACILITIES
Restrooms

🚶 DESTINATIONS	LENGTH	VERTICAL FEET	DIFFICULTY
WITH WATER TAXI	8.0 miles, 4 hours	±1,190	– 1 2 **3** 4 5 +
WITHOUT WATER TAXI	13.0 miles, 7 hours	±2,090	– 1 2 3 **4** 5 +

Hikers with rudimentary cross-country skills have a fantastic playground in the nooks and crannies of this alpinelike basin.

this road for 0.9 mile to the large trailhead parking area above the south shore of Lower Echo Lake.

Logistics

The Echo Lake Chalet offers water taxi service from the resort's dock at the south end of Lower Echo Lake to the public dock at the far end of Upper Echo Lake, reducing the hiking distance by more than 2 miles. The normal season runs from the Fourth of July through Labor Day weekend, though service usually extends through September depending on weather conditions and lake levels. At the time of research, the fee was $12 per person, one way, with a $36 per boatload minimum (dogs are $5 each). A direct phone line from the upper dock to the chalet can be used to arrange for pickup. When the channel to the upper lake is no longer navigable, usually by mid-September, passengers are dropped at the end of the lower lake for a reduced fee with a four-person minimum. Call 530-659-7207 (8 a.m.–6 p.m., summer only) for more information, or visit the website at **echochalet.com.**

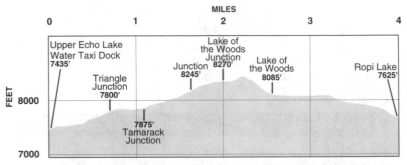

TRAIL 35   Echo Lake to Lake of the Woods & Ropi Lake Elevation Profile

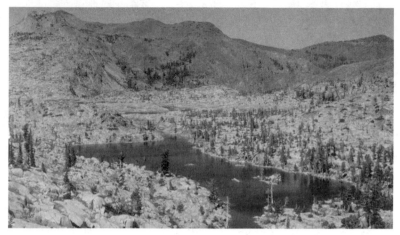

Ropi Lake

Trail Description

Without water taxi service, you'll have to walk the extra 2.5 miles around the north shore of Echo Lakes and add that distance to the following mileages. ►1 From the water taxi pier, climb to the junction with the Pacific Crest Trail (PCT). ►2 Turn left (west) and proceed on rocky tread across open slopes on a westbound course away from the lakes. Near the Desolation Wilderness boundary, 0.7 mile from the pier, you meet a junction with a lightly used trail to Triangle Lake. ►3 Another 0.4 mile of hiking leads to another junction, this one with a lateral to Tamarack, Ralston, and Cagwin Lakes. ►4 These three picturesque lakes are worth a visit if you have the extra time and energy.

Beyond the junction, the PCT follows a moderate climb to a diminutive rivulet coursing through a ravine and then continues the ascent via a pair of switchbacks to an open bench and a junction with the Tamarack Trail, 1.1 miles from the pier. ►5

 Lake

Wildflowers

Gently ascending trail brings you along the northern fringe of the broad expanse of grassy Haypress Meadows, where early- to midsummer wildflowers put on a fine floral display. Near the far end of the meadows, at 2.0 miles, is the junction with Trail 17E40 to Lake of the Woods. ►6

Leave the PCT and head southwest skirting the edge of Haypress Meadows and climbing to the crest of a low ridge, where you cross the Ralston Peak Trail. ►7 From the ridge, follow a moderately steep switchbacking descent to a junction near the northeast shore of Lake of the Woods, 2.6 miles from the Echo Lake pier. ►8

To reach Ropi Lake, head south along the east shore of Lake of the Woods and make a brief climb over the lip of the basin. On descending trail, you head down the canyon of the outlet to a crossing of the stream, at 3.5 miles. Follow the trail as it bends west and descends around a knob to the east shore of Ropi Lake. ►9 From there, the backcountry is your oyster, but make sure you pack a good topographic map and the requisite cross-country skills.

			MILESTONES
►1	0.0	2.5	Start at Upper Echo Lake pier
►2	0.1	2.6	Turn left (west) at PCT junction
►3	0.7	3.2	Continue straight ahead at Triangle Lake junction
►4	1.1	3.6	Continue straight ahead at Tamarack Lake junction
►5	1.7	4.2	Continue straight ahead at Tamarack Trail junction
►6	2.0	4.5	Turn left (southwest) at Lake of the Woods junction
►7	2.25	4.75	Continue straight ahead at Ralston Peak junction
►8	2.6	5.1	Lake of the Woods
►9	4.0	6.5	Ropi Lake

Ralston Peak

Though the climb is steady and stiff, where else in the Tahoe Basin can you achieve such a grand view with only a 3-mile hike? Most hikers favor the route to Ralston Peak from Echo Lakes, which is a mile longer via the water taxi (3.5 miles longer without) but requires 800 fewer feet of elevation gain. This being the case, you may not have to share the serenity of the route described below with too many other hikers.

Best Time

Snow has melted from the peak by mid- to late July, when wildflowers are at their peak. By the middle or end of October, Ralston Peak has usually seen the first snowfall of the season.

Finding the Trail

Drive US 50 to Sayles Flat and turn north onto a gravel and dirt road opposite the entrance into Camp Sacramento (about 5.75 miles west of Echo Summit and 1.25 miles east of Twin Bridges). Follow this road past the Chapel of Our Lady of the Sierra to the small parking area, 250 yards from the highway. If parking is not available at the trailhead, park along the broad shoulder of the highway at Sayles Flat.

Trail Description

▶1 The Ralston Peak Trail starts climbing right off the bat through the cool shade of a dense fir forest, where an occasional chinquapin shrub steals enough sunlight to eke out an existence. The trail snakes up the

TRAIL USE
Hike, Run,
Dogs Allowed

LENGTH
6.0 miles, 5 hours

VERTICAL FEET
±2,875

DIFFICULTY
– 1 2 3 **4** 5 +

TRAIL TYPE
Out-and-back

SURFACE TYPE
Dirt

FEATURES
Canyon
Mountain
Summit
Wildflowers
Birds
Great Views
Photo Opportunity
Steep
Secluded

FACILITIES
None

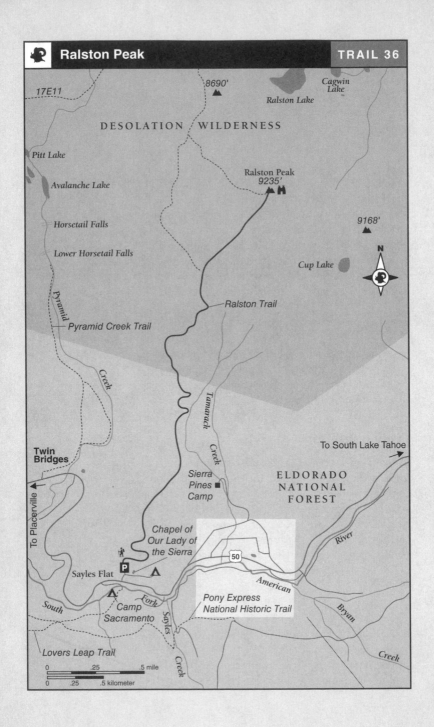

17E11

8690'

Cagwin Lake

Ralston Lake

DESOLATION   WILDERNESS

Pitt Lake

Avalanche Lake

Ralston Peak
9235'

9168'

Horsetail Falls

Lower Horsetail Falls

Cup Lake

N

Pyramid

Ralston Trail

Pyramid Creek Trail

Creek

Tamarack

Creek

To South Lake Tahoe

Twin
Bridges

Sierra
Pines
Camp

ELDORADO
NATIONAL
FOREST

To Placerville

Chapel of
Our Lady of
the Sierra

50

River

Sayles Flat

P

American

Sayles

Fork

Pony Express
National Historic Trail

South

Camp
Sacramento

Bryan

Lovers Leap Trail

Creek

Creek

0   .25   .5 mile

0   .25   .5 kilometer

hillside on a steady climb toward the huge moraine that forms the east lip of Pyramid Creek canyon, flirting with the possibility of a view into the deep gorge but failing to deliver until you've logged the first mile. At that point, a short use trail wanders to the brink of the canyon, where a fine vista unfolds.

A splendid view of Desolation Wilderness is at your feet.

Soon the trail makes a very brief descent to follow alongside a lushly lined stretch of Tamarack Creek, where alders, ferns, and scattered wildflowers interrupt the otherwise dry surroundings. All too soon the trail forsakes the creek and returns to a winding ascent of the morainal ridge, as a lighter forest allows chinquapin, manzanita, and huckleberry oak to flourish. Near the 1.5-mile mark, you uneventfully cross the unsigned boundary into Desolation Wilderness and follow a switchbacking climb into more open forest, where shrubs and boulders dot the slope. Views of the surrounding terrain improve with the gain in elevation, and you get glimpses of Pyramid Peak, Lovers Leap, and the ski runs of Sierra-at-Tahoe ski resort. After stepping over a boggy stretch of trail wet from a tiny seep spilling across the path, you continue the ascent across dry, meadowlike slopes, carpeted with lupine, asters, and mule-ears, to an unsigned junction, 2.25 miles from the trailhead. ▶2

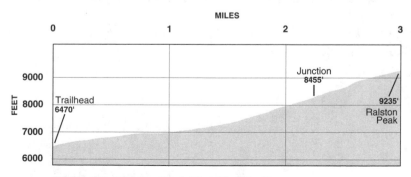

TRAIL 36 Ralston Peak Elevation Profile

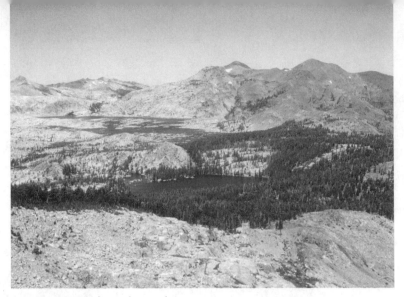

Desolation Valley *from Ralston Peak*

Leave the Ralston Peak Trail and follow the faint track of a ducked path that steeply climbs the southwest ridge of Ralston Peak through scattered western white pines and red firs. Higher up the slope, you pass a colorful, spring-fed patch of grasses and wildflowers before a final climb over fractured rocks **Summit** ▲ leads to the summit. ▶3 A splendid view of Desolation Wilderness is at your feet. More distant views include part of Lake Tahoe and the Freel Peak area.

🚶	**MILESTONES**	
▶1	0.0	Start at trailhead
▶2	2.25	Turn right (northeast) at use trail junction
▶3	3.0	Summit of Ralston Peak

Horsetail Falls

Tumbling down the head of the deep, ice-sculpted granite cleft of Pyramid Creek canyon, the thin ribbon of Horsetail Falls is dramatically scenic at any time of year, but especially spectacular during the height of snowmelt. Located a mere 1.5 miles from a major highway linking the Sacramento Valley with Lake Tahoe, conditions are ripe for this area to become very popular with both recreationists and sightseers alike. Parking improvements and construction of a short loop trail have made the area even more attractive.

Best Time

Horsetail Falls is most magnificent during the height of snowmelt, usually mid-June–mid-July. However, several deaths have occurred here over the years, and extreme caution should be exercised, especially when the rocks along Pyramid Creek are slick from spray. Families should keep a constant watch over young children.

Finding the Trail

Drive US 50 to Twin Bridges, approximately 6.75 miles west of Echo Summit, and park in the well-marked Pyramid Creek parking lot ($5 day-use fee, $20 annual fee). The trailhead area is complete with flush toilets and running water.

TRAIL USE
Hike
LENGTH
3.0 miles, 1.5 hours
VERTICAL FEET
±675
DIFFICULTY
– 1 2 **3** 4 5 +
TRAIL TYPE
Out-and-back
SURFACE TYPE
Dirt

FEATURES
Canyon
Mountain
Stream
Waterfall
Great Views
Photo Opportunity
Geologic Interest

FACILITIES
Restrooms
Picnic Tables
Water

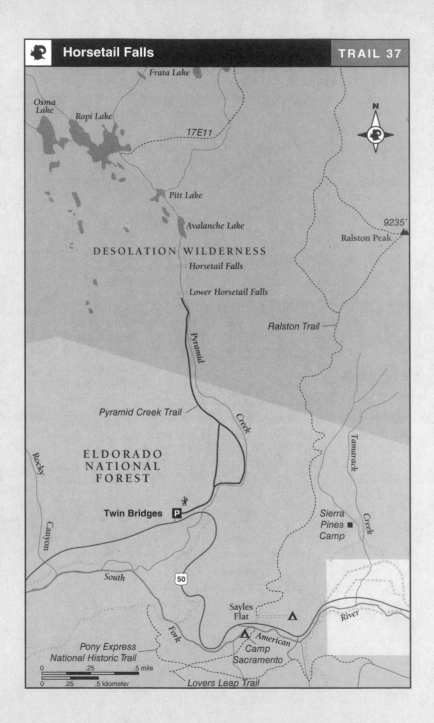

Frata Lake

Osma
Lake

Ropi Lake

17E11

Pitt Lake

Avalanche Lake

9235'

Ralston Peak

DESOLATION WILDERNESS

Horsetail Falls

Lower Horsetail Falls

Ralston Trail

Pyramid

Pyramid Creek Trail

Creek

ELDORADO
NATIONAL
FOREST

Rocky

Tamarack

Creek

Twin Bridges P

Sierra
Pines ■
Camp

Canyon

South

50

Sayles
Flat

River

Fork

American
Camp
Sacramento

Pony Express
National Historic Trail

0   .25   .5 mile
0   .25   .5 kilometer

Lovers Leap Trail

Logistics

Wilderness permits are required for overnight use. Overnight wilderness permit holders do not have to pay an additional day-use parking fee.

Trail Description

▶1 From the parking lot, follow singletrack trail through oaks, incense cedars, white firs, and Jeffrey pines, with an understory of chinquapin, huckleberry oak, and manzanita, to a trail junction near an area of large, sloping granite slabs. ▶2 Turn right (east), obeying a sign marked PYRAMID CREEK LOOP, CASCADE VISTA. Follow hiker emblem signs attached to widely spaced conifers as you hike over granite slabs alongside the twisting and turning course of Pyramid Creek, which tumbles over steps and swirls through cataracts. Continue climbing up the canyon, with occasional views of Horsetail Falls, following a route that alternates rock slabs with sections of dirt trail, progressing in and out of scattered forest. You veer away from the creek slightly and reach a junction, 0.75 mile from the trailhead. ▶3

To continue toward the falls, turn right (northwest) at the junction and hike over more slabs and sandy sections of trail to the signed Desolation

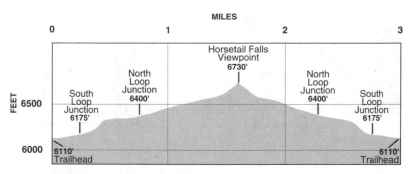

TRAIL 37 Horsetail Falls Elevation Profile

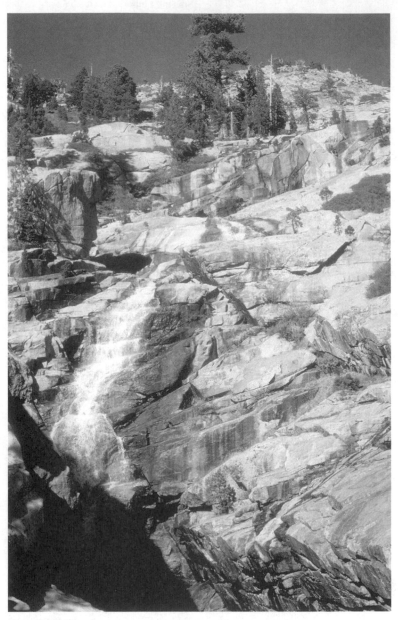

Horsetail Falls

Wilderness boundary and a day hikers' trail register just beyond. Proceed up the canyon a fair distance, away from the roaring creek through sparse stands of junipers and pines and patches of shrubs. Nearing the falls, the canyon narrows and the terrain becomes much steeper, forcing the rocky trail closer to the creek. Eventually, defined tread falters altogether as granite slabs and boulders bar the way. A short climb leads to a pool near the base of the lower falls, the turnaround point for most parties, especially in early season when the water-polished bedrock above is wet and slippery. ▶4

Though a well-known cross-country route continues up the canyon toward Desolation Valley, only skilled off-trail enthusiasts should contemplate this route.

You can streamline your return to the trailhead by following the Pyramid Creek Trail past the junctions with the Pyramid Creek Loop ▶5, ▶6 directly back to the parking lot. ▶7

The thin ribbon of Horsetail Falls is dramatically scenic at any time of year.

 Waterfall

🚶 MILESTONES

▶		
▶1	0.0	Start at trailhead
▶2	0.25	Turn right (east) at lower Pyramid Creek Loop junction
▶3	0.75	Turn right (northwest) at junction with Pyramid Creek Trail
▶4	1.5	Base of Lower Horsetail Falls
▶5	2.25	Continue straight ahead at upper Pyramid Creek Loop junction
▶6	2.75	Continue straight ahead at lower Pyramid Creek Loop junction
▶7	3.0	Return to trailhead

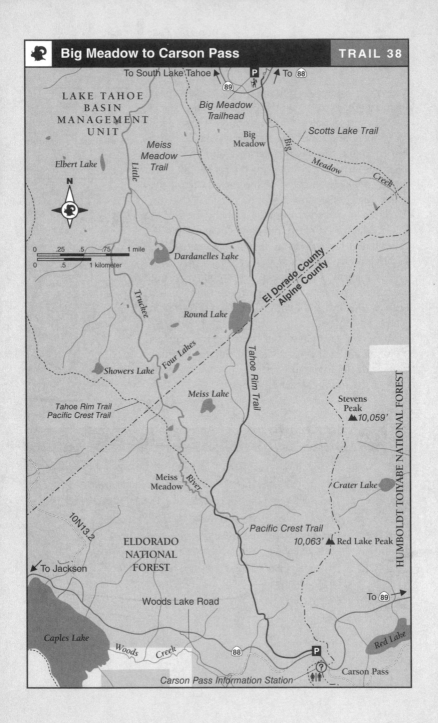

To South Lake Tahoe

To 88

P

89

Big Meadow
Trailhead

Big
Meadow

Scotts Lake Trail

LAKE TAHOE
BASIN
MANAGEMENT
UNIT

Meiss
Meadow
Trail

Elbert Lake

Big

Meadow

Creek

N

Little

0   .25   .5   .75   1 mile

0   .5   1 kilometer

Dardanelles Lake

El Dorado County
Alpine County

Truckee

Round Lake

Four Lakes

Tahoe Rim Trail

Showers Lake

Meiss Lake

Stevens
Peak
▲10,059'

HUMBOLDT TOIYABE NATIONAL FOREST

Tahoe Rim Trail
Pacific Crest Trail

Meiss
Meadow

River

Crater Lake

10N13.2

Pacific Crest Trail
10,063' ▲ Red Lake Peak

To Jackson

ELDORADO
NATIONAL
FOREST

To 89

Woods Lake Road

Caples Lake

Woods   Creek

88

Red Lake

P

?

Carson Pass

Carson Pass Information Station

Big Meadow to Carson Pass

With arrangements for a shuttle, a nearly 8-mile trip travels through the heart of the proposed 31,100-acre Meiss Meadow Wilderness. Following sections of the Tahoe Rim and Pacific Crest Trails, recreationists can travel from CA 89 to CA 88, visiting Big Meadow, Round Lake, and Meiss Meadows along the way. A 1.3-mile side trip to scenic Dardanelles Lake provides a fine diversion.

Best Time

Snow melts around the first of July and the wildflower season starts shortly thereafter, lasting until around mid-August. Autumn is a fine time to hike this trail, as aspens and meadow grasses turn golden and the number of trail users drops considerably.

Finding the Trail

The drive between the trailheads is roughly 16 miles.

START: Drive on CA 89 to the well-signed Tahoe Rim Trail parking lot, 6 miles from the CA 88 junction in Hope Valley, and 5 miles from the US 50 junction near Myers.

END: Follow CA 88 to the Meiss Meadows Trailhead parking lot, 0.2 mile west of Carson Pass.

Trail Description

▶1 Leave the parking area and follow the singletrack Tahoe Rim Trail (TRT) a short distance south to a crossing of CA 89. Once across the highway, start a

---

TRAIL USE
Hike, Run, Horses,
Dogs Allowed

LENGTH
10.4 miles, 6 hours

VERTICAL FEET
+2,075/-1,000

DIFFICULTY
− 1 2 **3** 4 5 +

TRAIL TYPE
Point-to-point

SURFACE TYPE
Dirt

FEATURES
Canyon
Mountain
Stream
Lake
Autumn Colors
Wildflowers
Birds
Wildlife
Photo Opportunity
Camping
Secluded
Historical Interest

FACILITIES
Restrooms

winding, moderate climb through a forest of Jeffrey pines, lodgepole pines, and red firs. At a switchback you have a fine view of the aspen-lined, rocky channel of Big Meadow Creek, which is alive with snowmelt in early July and golden color in autumn. Following more switchbacks, the grade eases just before reaching a three-way junction, 0.5 mile from the trailhead, where a trail to Scott Lake branches left. ▶2

Veer right at the junction and quickly leave the trees behind, as you emerge into the grassy, flower-covered clearing of Big Meadow. Follow the trail through the meadow to a wood-plank bridge that spans the gurgling creek, and proceed to the far edge, where a lightly forested ascent resumes.

Wildflowers Sagebrush, currant, and drought-tolerant wildflowers, principally mule-ears, line the path. Farther up the trail, wood-beam reinforced steps ameliorate the steeper sections of trail, alongside a diminishing tributary of Big Meadow Creek, a sprightly watercourse lined with luxuriant foliage. Continue climbing to a densely forested saddle, and then follow a switchbacking descent into the next canyon, through which flows an Upper Truckee River tributary. Reach the canyon floor and a three-way junction marked by an 8- by 8-inch post, where you meet the Meiss Meadows Trail, at 2.2 miles. ▶3

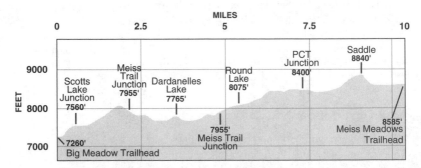

TRAIL 38 Big Meadow to Carson Pass Elevation Profile

From the Meiss Meadows Trail junction, head northwest for 0.2 mile to another three-way junction. ►4 Turn left (west), make a very brief descent to a boulder hop of the Upper Truckee River tributary, and soon encounter a ford of a wider stretch of the stream. Early in the season, you may need to search for logs upstream in order to make the second crossing without getting your feet wet. Away from the streams, stroll across a bench holding a small meadow and seasonal ponds. Descend off the bench, through dense forest of western white pines, red firs, and lodgepole pines, and follow an alder- and willow-lined stream down a canyon. The grade eases as you pass through meadowlike vegetation of grasses, wildflowers, and willows to the boulder hop of Round Lake's outlet. A short climb amid boulders and granite slabs leads to the west shore of Dardanelles Lake, 1.3 miles from the TRT. ►5

Far enough off the thoroughfare of the TRT, you may be able to enjoy the relative seclusion of this lake. The lakeshore is shaded by light forest and dotted with boulders and slabs, and the picturesque cliffs of the Dardanelles loom above the south shore.

When you're ready, return to the Meiss Meadows Trail junction. The route of the TRT follows a steady climb through dense forest. After 0.6 mile, you reach the lip of Round Lake's basin above the northeast shore and also an informal junction. ►6 From the junction a use trail wraps around the lake's west shore, which is lined with rock outcrops and scattered forest, and then follows a cross-country route to Meiss Lake. The TRT skirts the east shore of Round Lake through thick forest, away from the lush meadows and thick willows that border the inlet at the south end.

Beyond the lake the TRT resumes its climbing ways, soon reaching an extensive, sloping meadow carpeted with willows, wildflowers, and other lush foliage, which is well watered by a thin, rock-lined

Autumn is a fine time to hike this trail, as aspens and meadow grasses turn golden.

 Lake

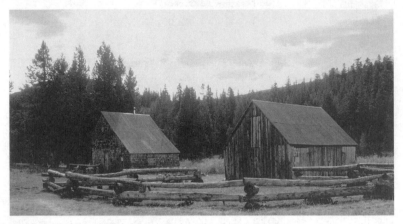

Historical cabins *along the Upper Truckee River in Meiss Meadows*

rivulet spilling across the trail. Away from the meadow, you reenter forest cover and hop across a pair of trickling rivulets. Eventually the grade eases to a mellow stroll as you break out into an open forest sprinkled with stands of aspen and swaths of drier ground cover, which includes sagebrush, currant, grasses, and drought-tolerant wildflowers.

A part of the extensive network of Meiss Meadows appears through scattered lodgepole pines to the right of the trail, with Meiss Lake lying just one-third mile to the west. Leaving the meadow behind, you hop across Round Lake's inlet and proceed to the crossing of a creek coursing through a rocky channel, 0.4 mile farther on. Here, open terrain allows views of the rugged slopes leading up to 10,059-foot Stevens Peak. Continue on gently graded trail through lodgepole pines to the heart of Meiss Meadows and a well-signed junction with the Pacific Crest Trail (PCT), 7.7 miles from the trailhead. ▶7

Historical Interest

Near the junction, an old cabin harks back to the days, not so long ago, when cattle were allowed to graze the lush grasses of picturesque and pastoral Meiss Meadows. Fortunately, the cows are gone, the trampling of the meadows is over, the cow pies have decomposed, and the trails have been left to the bipeds. Heading south on the PCT from the junction, stroll across the pleasant meadowlands to a crossing

Red Lake Peak

OPTION

Peak baggers with extra time and energy could accept the challenge of climbing Red Lake Peak from the saddle, 1.2 miles northwest of the Meiss Meadows Trailhead. ▶8 A bit of history: John C. Frémont and Charles Pruess reached the summit on Valentine's Day in 1844 and were the first Europeans to record a sighting of Lake Tahoe.

of the Upper Truckee River and follow it upstream to a second crossing. Soon afterward, the terrain gets steeper and you start a moderate climb of a narrowing gorge to a saddle at the head of the canyon just beyond a seasonal pond, 9.2 miles from the trailhead. ▶8 From here, enjoy a fine view to the south of the jagged peaks of the Carson Pass area.

 Great Views

Leaving the saddle, you make a steep 0.3-mile descent across a stream and into light forest, followed by an arcing traverse across the hillside above CA 88. At 10.4 miles, you reach the Meiss Meadows Trailhead. ▶9

🚶	MILESTONES	
▶1	0.0	Start at Big Meadow Trailhead
▶2	0.5	Veer right at junction with Scotts Lake Trail
▶3	2.2	Turn right (northwest) at Meiss Meadows Trail junction
▶4	2.4	Turn left (west) at Dardanelles Lake junction
▶5	3.5	Dardanelles Lake
▶4	4.6	Return to Dardanelles Lake junction; turn right (east)
▶3	4.8	Return to Meiss Meadows Trail junction; turn right (southeast)
▶6	5.4	Round Lake
▶7	7.7	Turn left (south) at PCT junction
▶8	9.2	Saddle with views of Carson Pass
▶9	10.4	Reach Meiss Meadows Trailhead

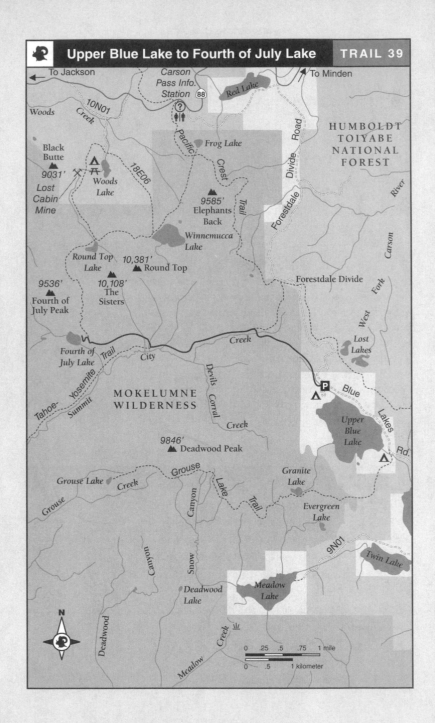

To Jackson

Carson Pass Info. Station 88

To Minden

Red Lake

Woods

10N01 Creek

HUMBOLDT TOIYABE NATIONAL FOREST

Black Butte

9031'

Lost Cabin Mine

Woods Lake

18E06

Pacific

Frog Lake

Divide Road

Forestdale

Carson River

9585' Elephants Back

Crest

West Fork

Winnemucca Lake

Round Top Lake

10,381' Round Top

Trail

Forestdale Divide

9536' Fourth of July Peak

10,108' The Sisters

Lost Lakes

Creek

Fourth of July Lake

Summit

City

Tahoe-Yosemite Trail

MOKELUMNE WILDERNESS

Devils Corral

P

Blue

Creek

Lakes

9846' Deadwood Peak

Grouse

Upper Blue Lake

Rd.

Grouse Lake

Creek

Lake

Canyon

Trail

Granite Lake

Evergreen Lake

Grouse

Snow

9N01

Twin Lake

Canyon

Deadwood Lake

Meadow Lake

Creek

N

Deadwood

Meadow

| 0 | .25 | .5 | .75 | 1 mile |

| 0 | | .5 | | 1 kilometer |

Upper Blue Lake to Fourth of July Lake

This route from Upper Blue Lake is definitely the back way to Fourth of July Lake because most visitors reach the lake from either the Woods Lake or Carson Pass Trailheads near CA 88. The advantage to this route is not limited to the potential for solitude alone, as views of Summit City Canyon and the neighboring peaks are quite remarkable.

Best Time

The snow-free season usually begins mid-July and runs through mid-October.

Finding the Trail

Leave CA 88 at 6.3 miles east of Carson Pass and head south on Blue Lakes Road through the southern part of Hope Valley and over a divide to a junction with the Tamarack Road, 10.3 miles from CA 88. Continue straight ahead and proceed for another mile and then turn right at the Mokelumne Hydro Project. Proceed past Lower Blue Lake and Upper Blue Lake to the signed Evergreen Trailhead 18E21 on the right-hand side of the road, just prior to the entrance to Upper Blue Lake Campground. Limited parking is available at the trailhead.

Logistics

A wilderness permit is required for overnight use. Camping at Fourth of July Lake is limited to designated sites only. Permits can be obtained at the information center at Carson Pass.

TRAIL USE
Hike, Horses,
Dogs Allowed
LENGTH
9.0 miles, 5 hours
VERTICAL FEET
±1,150
DIFFICULTY
– 1 2 3 **4** 5 +
TRAIL TYPE
Out-and-back
SURFACE TYPE
Dirt

FEATURES
Canyon
Lake
Wildflowers
Birds
Wildlife
Great Views
Photo Opportunity
Camping

FACILITIES
Restrooms

Trail Description

▶1 Begin hiking on an old roadbed on a moderate climb through a mixed forest of white firs, lodgepole pines, western white pines, and mountain hemlocks alongside the thin, alder-lined inlet of Upper Blue Lake. Cross the narrow creek and continue upstream along the east bank to a small meadow **Wildflowers** 🌼 filled with brilliant wildflowers in midsummer, before soon returning to dense forest cover. Eventually the trail moves away from the diminutive stream and crosses the signed Mokelumne Wilderness boundary. Beyond the boundary, the grade of ascent increases for a short distance on the way to the top of a ridge, beyond which your descent into Summit City Canyon begins.

Initially, the descent into the canyon is fairly steep, but soon moderates on the approach to a crossing of Summit City Creek, which occurs just above the lip of a short waterfall. Just past the crossing is an obscure three-way junction with a trail climbing northeast toward Forestdale Divide.

Follow the creek downstream through the deep canyon. Occasional, filtered views through the trees of Deadwood Peak across the chasm of Summit City Canyon provide intriguing glimpses of some

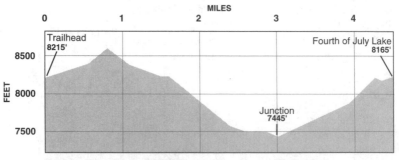

TRAIL 39 Upper Blue Lake to Fourth of July Lake Elevation Profile

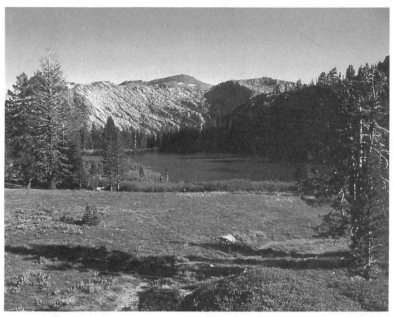

Fourth of July Lake

alpine-looking terrain that seems deserving of a fuller view. Soon the tread becomes rocky and steep, as the forest lightens a bit, which allows a healthy ground cover of sagebrush, grasses, and drought-tolerant wildflowers to flourish. The dry foliage is briefly interrupted by a lushly lined seep trickling across the trail. Beyond the seep, the ground cover is diminished by dense forest. Farther on, a break in the trees allows the fuller view of Deadwood Peak for which you may have previously longed.

Continue the moderate descent on rocky tread through thick forest until the grade eases on the approach to the bottom of the canyon, where meadowlike vegetation carpets the forest floor. A gentle stroll then leads past a primitive campsite to a 4- by 4-inch post marking the junction of a trail on the right to Fourth of July Lake, 3.0 miles from the trailhead. ▶2

Turn right (north) and start a moderate climb that leads out of the forest cover and onto shrub-covered slopes. Soon the trail bends west to follow a rising traverse across the open hillside, where the trail is nearly overgrown in places by the thick shrubs. Fine views of Summit City Canyon and Deadwood and Fourth of July Peaks abound on this rising ascent. Nearing the steep canyon of the outlet from Fourth of July Lake, the trail veers northeast and switchbacks into scattered forest and crosses the boundary of the Carson Pass Management Area. Additional switchbacks then lead to the east shore of Fourth of July Lake. ▶3

Lake

Reposing in the cirque at the base of a peak of the same name, Fourth of July Lake is rimmed by steep cliffs, stands of forest, patches of willow, and pockets of flower-filled meadow. Camping is limited to the six designated sites available by reservation only on the east and north sides of the lake.

Camping ⛺

🚶	MILESTONES	
▶1	0.0	Start at trailhead
▶2	3.0	Turn right at junction to Fourth of July Lake
▶3	4.5	Fourth of July Lake

Winnemucca and Round Top Lakes Loop

Two picturesque, near timberline lakes with a stunning backdrop from the craggy summits of The Sisters and Round Top are the chief attractions of this loop. The wildflower displays along the upper canyons of Woods Creek are quite colorful in season. Views of the Lost Cabin Mine add a touch of historical interest. Additional options for extending the journey include a 2.3-mile hike to Fourth of July Lake or a technically easy climb of Round Top.

Best Time

The Carson Pass region, with elevations over 8,000 feet, tends to hold onto its mantle of snow well into the summer, especially after winters of heavy snowfall. Though mid-July may see trails open up in some years, late July is a better bet following an average winter. Wildflowers are at their peak July–mid-August. Mild daytime temperatures usually continue until the end of September and, though cooler, autumn hiking can be quite pleasant until the first major storm, usually toward the end of October.

Finding the Trail

Follow CA 88 to the access road for Woods Lake, 1.7 miles west of Carson Pass. Follow the paved access road for 0.8 mile to a junction and turn right, driving another 0.1 mile to the Woods Lake Trailhead parking lot, which has a pit toilet.

TRAIL USE
Hike, Run, Horses, Dogs Allowed

LENGTH
4.8 miles, 2–3 hours

VERTICAL FEET
±1,200

DIFFICULTY
– 1 2 **3** 4 5 +

TRAIL TYPE
Loop

SURFACE TYPE
Dirt

FEATURES
Canyon
Mountain
Stream
Lake
Wildflowers
Photo Opportunity
Camping
Historical Interest

FACILITIES
Restrooms
Picnic Tables
Water
Campground

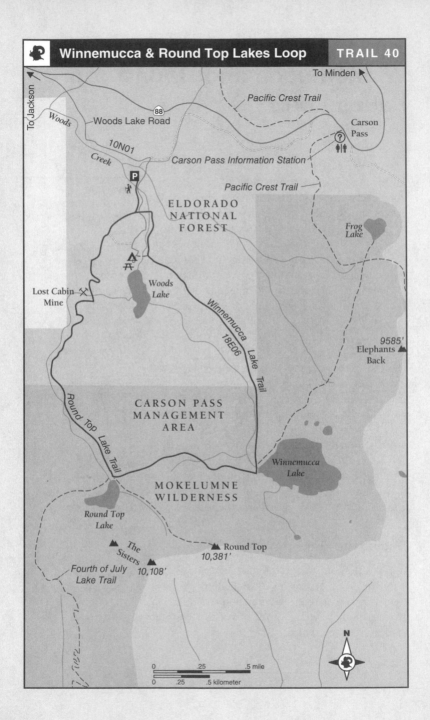

Winnemucca & Round Top Lakes Loop

TRAIL 40

To Minden

Pacific Crest Trail

To Jackson

Woods

Woods Lake Road

88

10N01

Creek

Carson Pass Information Station

Carson Pass

P

Pacific Crest Trail

ELDORADO NATIONAL FOREST

Frog Lake

Lost Cabin Mine

Woods Lake

Winnemucca Lake Trail

18E06

9585'
Elephants Back

CARSON PASS MANAGEMENT AREA

Round Top Lake Trail

Winnemucca Lake

MOKELUMNE WILDERNESS

Round Top Lake

The Sisters

Round Top
10,381'

Fourth of July Lake Trail

10,108'

0   .25   .5 mile

0   .25   .5 kilometer

N

Logistics

A wilderness permit is required for overnight use. Camping at Winnemucca, Round Top, and Fourth of July Lakes is limited to designated sites only. Permits can be obtained at the information center at Carson Pass.

The wildflower displays along the upper canyons of Woods Creek are quite colorful in season.

Trail Description

►1 From the parking lot, walk a short distance along the access road across a bridge to the start of the Round Top Lake Trail (17E47). Proceed on dirt trail through a mixed forest of white firs, mountain hemlocks, and western white pines and soon come above the access road to Woods Lake Campground. Reaching a junction, you proceed to the right, following a sign for Round Top Lake. A short, moderate climb leads above the campground, where the singletrack trail merges with an old road. Follow the road on a moderate, winding climb to the Lost Cabin Mine Trailhead, 0.5 mile from the parking lot.

 Camping

Back on singletrack trail, climb amid scattered trees with a filtered view of Round Top to the southeast and Woods Lake below. After hopping across boulder- and willow-lined Woods Creek, you follow

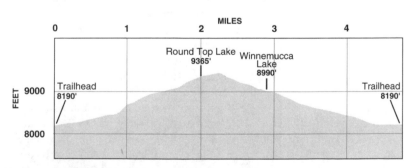

TRAIL 40 Winnemucca & Round Top Lakes Loop Elevation Profile

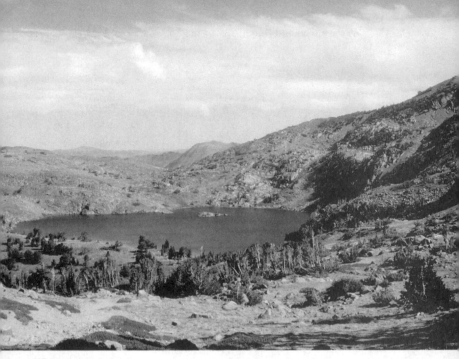

Winnemucca Lake

a switchbacking climb above the old structures of the Lost Cabin Mine. The mine was in operation until the early 1960s, producing copious quantities of gold, silver, copper, and lead.

Continue the ascent on a course roughly paralleling the west fork of Woods Creek. The grade eventually eases as you approach the wilderness boundary, and the volcanic summits of The Sisters and Round Top spring into view. Farther upstream, the canyon widens and you pass through open, subalpine terrain carpeted with clumps of willow, patches of heather, and wildflowers.

Nearing Round Top Lake, a 4- by 4-inch post marks a Y-junction with a trail to Fourth of July Lake, 2 miles from the parking lot. ▶2 You could follow the 2.3-mile trail on an hour-long trip to the lake easily enough, but make sure you save plenty of energy for the 2,300-foot climb back to the junction. Round Top Lake is a picturesque gem lined with stands of gnarled whitebark pines, dramatically backdropped by the dark, volcanic slopes of The Sisters and Round Top.

Great Views

From the Fourth of July junction, head east on a mildly rising climb over a granite ridge amid widely scattered, wind-battered whitebark pines and ground-hugging shrubs and grasses. From the crest of the ridge head down a gully on a moderate descent, cross the gully's stream and continue the descent through open terrain toward Winnemucca Lake. Nearing the lake, you cross the outlet on a flat-topped log and reach a 4- by 4-inch post at a three-way junction on the west shore, 2.9 miles from the trailhead. ▶3 Pockets of whitebark pine shelter designated campsites on the north shore of Winnemucca Lake, while dark cliffs rise up from the south shore, beneath the towering presence of Round Top. A mile to the northeast is the rounded hump of Elephant's Back.

Camping

From the junction, a 1.4-mile trail ascends the slope below Elephant's Back to a connection near Frog Lake with the Pacific Crest Trail, which then

OPTION

Side Trip to Round Top

Ambitious adventurers with plenty of extra energy could accept the challenge of a summit bid on the 10,381-foot peak by following a boot-beaten path up the gully of the lake's inlet toward the saddle between east Sister and Round Top. Before reaching the saddle, the route veers into a distinct notch in a ridge and then follows the ridge toward a false summit. Many parties are content with reaching the false summit as their destination, as the true summit is not much higher and requires some exposed scrambling to reach. As expected, the view from either summit is quite extraordinary. Exercise caution and good judgment on a climb of Round Top, and be prepared for windy conditions and intense sunlight at this altitude.

heads up another mile to Carson Pass. Your route veers to the north and follows the course of the east branch of Woods Creek, through mostly open terrain covered with sagebrush, willows, and an assortment of seasonal wildflowers. Leave the Mokelumne Wilderness a half mile from Winnemucca Lake and continue the steady descent into a light covering of mountain hemlocks. Nearing the trailhead, you pass a lateral to Woods Lake on the left, walk across a substantial wood bridge over the creek, cross the paved access road, and then return to the parking area. ▶4

🚶	MILESTONES	
▶1	0.0	Start at trailhead
▶2	2.0	Round Top Lake, proceed straight ahead at Fourth of July junction
▶3	2.9	Winnemucca Lake; veer left at Carson Pass junction
▶4	4.8	Return to trailhead

Emigrant Lake

Two lakes, one large and one small, provide hikers with two distinctly different portraits of the Carson Pass environs. More than half the journey follows the shoreline of Caples Lake, a 600-acre, man-made reservoir, where scads of recreationists boat, swim, and fish. The 4-mile trail ends at Emigrant Lake, a diminutive, natural lake filling the basin of a steep cirque rimmed by 9,500-foot-plus peaks.

Best Time

Dense forest cover along Emigrant Creek and the north-facing cirque containing Emigrant Lake provide cool conditions that inhibit any rapid melt of the previous winter's snowfall. Consequently, in average years you won't find a snow-free trail until mid-July. A brilliant floral display in the cirque will please wildflower enthusiasts from then until mid-August.

Finding the Trail

Drive CA 88 to the west end of Caples Lake and the large parking area near the dam.

Logistics

A wilderness permit is required for overnight visits.

Trail Description

►1 From the parking lot, the trail makes a very brief climb to a nice view of Caples Lake and follows the shoreline of the reservoir and the edge of the

TRAIL USE
Hike, Run, Horses,
Dogs Allowed

LENGTH
8.2 miles, 5 hours

VERTICAL FEET
+800/-25

DIFFICULTY
– 1 2 **3** 4 5 +

TRAIL TYPE
Out-and-back

SURFACE TYPE
Dirt

FEATURES
Canyon
Mountain
Stream
Lake
Wildflowers
Cool & Shady
Photo Opportunity
Camping

FACILITIES
Restrooms
Picnic Tables

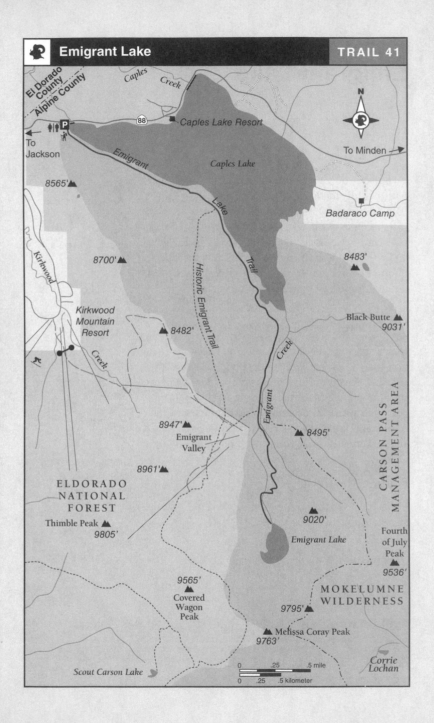

El Dorado
County
Alpine County

Caples Creek

88

Caples Lake Resort

N

To Minden →

To
Jackson

Emigrant

Caplcs Lake

Badaraco Camp

8565'▲

Kirkwood Creek

8700'▲

Lake

8483'

Historic Emigrant Trail

Trail

Black Butte ▲
9031'

Kirkwood
Mountain
Resort

▲ 8482'

Emigrant Creek

8947'▲▲
Emigrant
Valley

Emigrant Creek

▲ 8495'

8961'▲▲

CARSON PASS
MANAGEMENT AREA

ELDORADO
NATIONAL
FOREST

9020'▲

Thimble Peak ▲
9805'

Emigrant Lake

Fourth
of July
Peak
▲
9536'

9565'
▲
Covered
Wagon
Peak

MOKELUMNE
WILDERNESS

9795'▲

▲ Melissa Coray Peak
9763'

Corrie
Lochan

Scout Carson Lake

0   .25   .5 mile
0   .25   .5 kilometer

Mokelumne Wilderness on a virtually level course for the first 2.3 miles of your journey. A mixed forest of lodgepole pines, white firs, western white pines, and mountain hemlocks rims the lake, but because the trail stays so close to the lakeshore, you're guaranteed plenty of views across the lake of the surrounding cliffs, ridges, and peaks. Boaters on Caples Lake must observe a 5-mile-per-hour speed limit, which tends to keep engine noise to a minimum and helps to maintain the tranquility of the hike.

A brilliant floral display in the cirque will please wildflower enthusiasts.

Along the initial stretch of trail, you're apt to pass several anglers plying the water in search of a trophy-size trout. You then enter a more open area strewn with boulders and reach a signed junction with the Historic Emigrant Trail, 1.3 miles from the trailhead. ▶2 This old route eventually climbs to the crest of the ridge above Emigrant Lake between Covered Wagon and Melissa Coray Peaks.

Beyond the junction, follow the Emigrant Lake Trail back into the forest and continue the lakeshore stroll. Eventually the path moves farther away from the shoreline. Approaching Emigrant Creek, the trail veers south and begins a moderate climb up the forested canyon. Pass through a small meadow, where senecio and corn lily brighten the surroundings. Proceed upstream along the willow- and flower-lined creek to a signed T-junction, 3.0 miles from

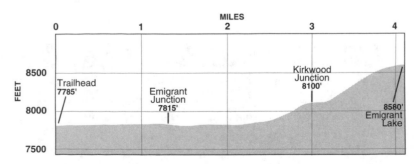

TRAIL 41 Emigrant Lake Elevation Profile

Caples Lake

HISTORY

Two small lakes known as Twin Lakes occupied this area before Pacific Gas and Electric dammed Caples Creek and created the Caples Lake Reservoir. The lake and creek were named for James Caples, a physician who in 1849 left Illinois with his family to join a wagon train bound for California. As a resident of California, Dr. Caples had stints as a miner and a merchant before managing a 4,000-acre ranch near Carson and Deer Creeks.

the trailhead, where a section of trail heads west to Kirkwood Meadows. ►3

About 0.1 mile beyond the junction, the trail crosses Emigrant Creek and climbs more steeply upstream to a set of switchbacks. Beyond the switchbacks, the grade eases and you stroll easily through thinning forest to the northeast shore of Emigrant Lake. ►4

Nestled in a deep north-facing cirque of steep cliffs with vertical walls holding lingering snowfields, Emigrant Lake has a cool, alpinelike ambiance, punctuated by the chilly winds that sweep across the surface of the lake. While a few clumps of trees and pockets of willows dot the near shore, most of the shoreline is stark and exposed, which only augments the unprotected feeling of the surroundings. However, the austere beauty of the area is quite stunning and you won't be disappointed with the scenery.

MILESTONES

►1	0.0	Start at trailhead
►2	1.3	Continue straight ahead at Historic Emigrant Trail junction
►3	3.0	Continue straight ahead at Kirkwood Meadows junction
►4	4.1	Emigrant Lake

Thunder Mountain

An incredible vista from a 9,408-foot summit should sound intriguing, especially if the trail to that summit is only 2.75 miles long, has an elevation gain less than 1,000 feet, and is accessible from a major highway. If that sounds too good to be true, think again, for such is the case with the Thunder Mountain Trail. Despite these positive attributes, the trail sees less use than you might imagine.

Best Time

The expansive view from the summit is good all the time, but getting there will be much easier once the trail becomes snow-free, usually toward the end of July. Good conditions usually extend through summer and into fall, until the first storm of the season drops significant snowfall on the Sierra, usually by late October.

Finding the Trail

Follow CA 88 to the roadside trailhead for the Thunder Mountain Loop near Carson Spur, 1.7 miles west of the Kirkwood Meadows junction.

Trail Description

▶1 Pass through a cattle gate in a wire fence, where you'll see a couple of trail signs, one with an ominous warning about unexploded ordnance used during winter for avalanche control. Proceed through a mixed forest of red firs, lodgepole pines, and western white pines, soon encountering a T-junction with a

TRAIL USE
Hike, Run, Bike,
Horses, Dogs Allowed

LENGTH
8.5 miles, 5 hours

VERTICAL FEET
+950/-300

DIFFICULTY
– 1 2 **3** 4 5 +

TRAIL TYPE
Out-and-back

SURFACE TYPE
Dirt

FEATURES
Mountain
Summit
Birds
Great Views
Photo Opportunity

FACILITIES
None

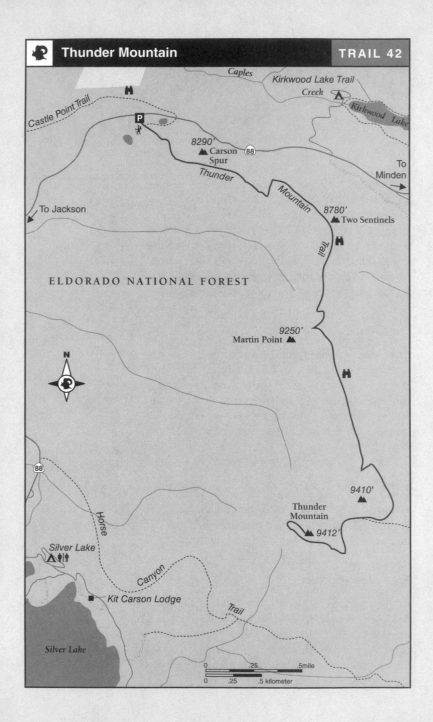

Thunder Mountain

TRAIL 42

Caples
Kirkwood Lake Trail
Creek
Kirkwood Lake

Castle Point Trail

P

8290'
Carson
Spur

88

To
Minden

Thunder

Mountain

8780'
Two Sentinels

To Jackson

ELDORADO NATIONAL FOREST

Trail

N

9250'
Martin Point

88

Horse

9410'

Thunder
Mountain

9412'

Silver Lake

Canyon

Kit Carson Lodge

Trail

Silver Lake

0		.25		.5 mile
0	.25		.5 kilometer	

lightly used path that heads east to cross CA 88 and
then west to Castle Point. ▶2 Continue straight ahead
on a moderate climb, breaking out of the trees as you
climb across a sagebrush- and wildflower-covered
hillside below Carson Spur, where the rocky crags of
Two Sentinels come into view. Briefly gain the crest
at a saddle before a climb across the west side of the
ridge leads into thickening forest. Following a pair
of switchbacks, you traverse below the pinnacles of
Two Sentinels to an open saddle, where the peaks
of the Carson Pass area burst into view, along with
Kirkwood Meadows and Caples Lake.

Head south along the ridge toward Martin Point,
enjoying additional eastward views along the way.
A couple of switchbacks lead to an upward traverse
around the east side of Martin Point, revealing the
impressive profile of Thunder Mountain's north
face, where the dark volcanic rock, punctuated
with clefts, gashes, pinnacles, and arêtes, creates a
dramatic alpine scene. Continue the ascent along
the ridge crest toward Thunder Mountain. As you
approach the northeast ridge of the peak, two more
switchbacks lead to a mild traverse around the back
of the ridge to a three-way junction, 3.5 miles from
the trailhead. ▶3

From the junction, veer to the right and follow
an ascending, westward traverse through scattered

**Thunder Mountain's
volcanic rock creates
a dramatic alpine
scene.**

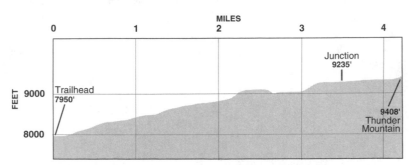

TRAIL 42 Thunder Mountain Elevation Profile

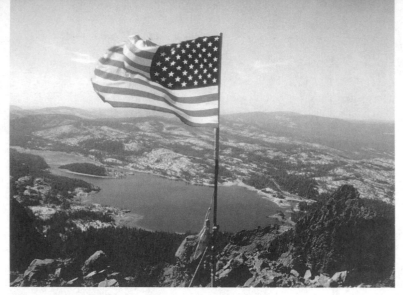

View *from Thunder Mountain*

lodgepole pines, western white pines, mountain hemlocks, and whitebark pines. The trees diminish as you reach the crest and then angle sharply to the east, following the ridge to the summit of Thunder Mountain. ▶4 An incredible view in all directions greets you at the top, from the mountains of northern Yosemite National Park in the south to the peaks of Desolation Wilderness in the north. Nearby landmarks include Silver and Caples Lakes and Round Top.

Great Views

MILESTONES

▶1	0.0	Start at trailhead
▶2	0.1	Proceed straight ahead at Castle Point junction
▶3	3.5	Turn right (southwest) at Thunder Mountain junction
▶4	4.25	Summit of Thunder Mountain

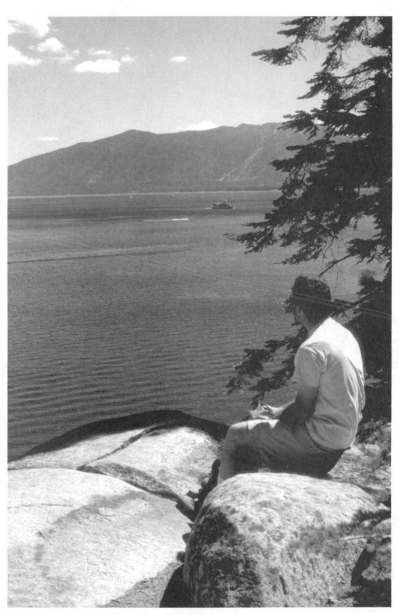

Lake Tahoe *from the Rubicon Trail (Trail 25)*

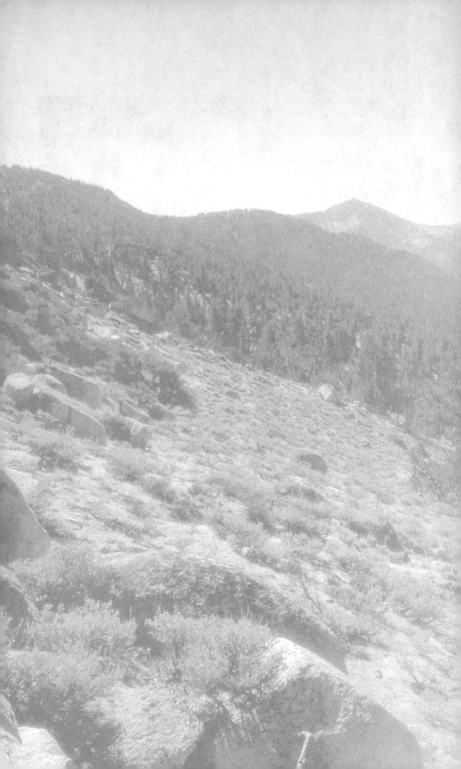

CHAPTER 4

East Tahoe

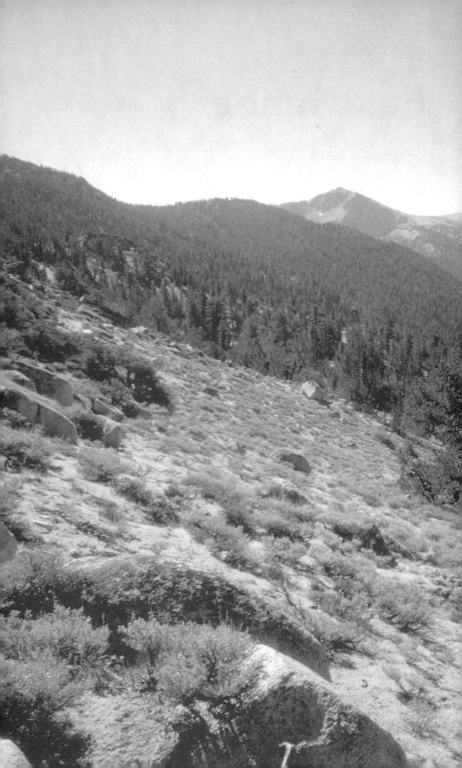

East Tahoe

The east side of the lake is perhaps the least developed area around Lake Tahoe. With such a distinction, the logical conclusion would be that this side of the lake would offer an abundance of backcountry trails. Ironically, until the relatively recent completion of the Tahoe Rim Trail (TRT), the area was considerably lacking in a developed and maintained trail system. Nowadays, with the building of the TRT and the closing of certain roadways in the backcountry of Lake Tahoe Nevada State Park to motorized travel, recreationists have plenty of opportunities to hike, bike, or ride in the mountainous terrain of east Tahoe.

Access to the forest lands is straightforward on two highways. The four-lane thoroughfare of US 50 climbs west to Spooner Summit from Carson City and then runs along the southeast shore of the lake before leaving the basin beyond South Lake Tahoe at Echo Summit. NV 28, from a junction with US 50, takes motorists northbound along the east shore and into California.

Permits and Maps

The backcountry on the lake's east side falls under the jurisdiction of three governing agencies, the Carson Ranger District of the Humboldt–Toiyabe National Forest, the Lake Tahoe Basin Management Unit of the federal government, and Lake Tahoe Nevada State Park. Without any designated wilderness areas, permits are not required for day hikes or backpacks. However, overnighters desiring to camp within the backcountry of Lake Tahoe Nevada State Park are restricted to designated campgrounds; call 775-831-0494 for reservations or more information. The park charges an entry fee.

U.S. Forest Service maps may be procured at ranger stations in Carson City and Truckee, or from the Taylor Creek Visitor Center. A full-color map

Opposite and overleaf: *Freel Peak area (Trail 50)*

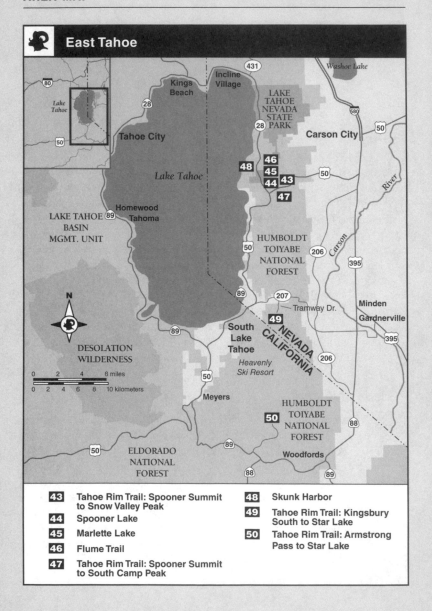

East Tahoe

43	Tahoe Rim Trail: Spooner Summit to Snow Valley Peak	**48**	Skunk Harbor
44	Spooner Lake	**49**	Tahoe Rim Trail: Kingsbury South to Star Lake
45	Marlette Lake	**50**	Tahoe Rim Trail: Armstrong Pass to Star Lake
46	Flume Trail		
47	Tahoe Rim Trail: Spooner Summit to South Camp Peak		

East Tahoe Trails

TRAIL	DIFFICULTY	LENGTH	TYPE	USES & ACCESS	TERRAIN	FLORA & FAUNA	EXPOSURE & OTHER
43	4	12.4					
44	1	1.8					
45	3	9.0					
46	3	13.0					
47	3	10.2					
48	3	3.2					
49	4	17.6					
50	3	12.8					

USES & ACCESS
- Day Hiking
- Running
- Mountain Biking
- Horses
- Dogs Allowed
- Child-Friendly
- Wheelchair Access
- Permit

TYPE
- Loop
- Out-and-back
- Point-to-point

DIFFICULTY
- 1 2 3 4 5 +
less   more

TERRAIN
- Canyon
- Mountain
- Summit
- Stream
- Waterfall
- Lake/Shore

FLORA & FAUNA
- Autumn Colors
- Wildflowers
- Birds
- Wildlife

EXPOSURE
- Cool & Shady
- Great Views
- Photo Opportunity

OTHER
- Camping
- Secluded
- Historical Interest
- Geologic Interest
- Steep

showing the backcountry routes of Lake Tahoe Nevada State Park is available at park headquarters near Spooner Lake, from state park headquarters in Carson City, or from the park's website at **parks.nv.gov/parks/marlette-hobart-backcountry.** USGS 7.5-minute quadrangles for trips covered in this section are listed in Appendix 4.

East Tahoe

Tahoe Rim Trail: Spooner Summit to South Camp Peak 297

One of the more lightly used sections of the Tahoe Rim Trail leads to a mile-long, continuous Lake Tahoe view from the broad summit of South Camp Peak.

TRAIL 47

Hike, Run, Bike, Horses, Dogs Allowed
10.2 miles,
Out-and-back
Difficulty: 1 2 **3** 4 5

Skunk Harbor 302

The sandy beaches of Lake Tahoe are world famous, and this trail keeps beach lovers to a manageable number with a 1.6-mile hike to a picturesque harbor, where a restored mansion offers a glimpse into the lake's resort era.

TRAIL 48

Hike, Run, Bike,
Child Friendly
3.2 miles, Out-and-back
Difficulty: 1 2 **3** 4 5

Tahoe Rim Trail: Kingsbury South to Star Lake 306

Along this section of the Tahoe Rim Trail, recreationists are treated to excellent views of Carson Valley and Lake Tahoe Basin before arriving at one of the area's highest lakes.

TRAIL 49

Hike, Run, Bike, Horses, Dogs Allowed
17.6 miles,
Out-and-back
Difficulty: 1 2 3 **4** 5

Tahoe Rim Trail: Armstrong Pass to Star Lake 311

The short route to beautiful Star Lake offers the bonus of standing on top of the Tahoe Basin's highest summit. Freel Peak, at 10,881 feet, offers a panoramic view of Tahoe and the hinterlands.

TRAIL 50

Hike, Run, Bike, Horses, Dogs Allowed
12.8 miles,
Out-and-back
Difficulty: 1 2 **3** 4 5

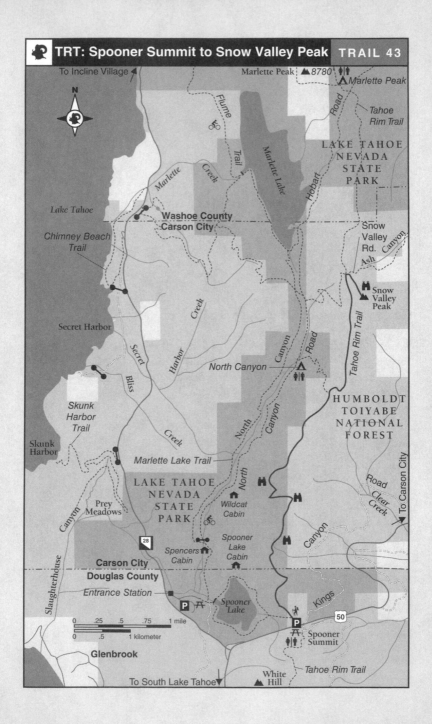

TRT: Spooner Summit to Snow Valley Peak · TRAIL 43

To Incline Village

N

Marlette Peak ▲ 8780

▲ Marlette Peak

Flume Trail

Marlette Lake

Hobart Road

Tahoe Rim Trail

LAKE TAHOE NEVADA STATE PARK

Marlette Creek

Lake Tahoe

Washoe County
Carson City

Snow Valley Rd.

Ash Canyon

Chimney Beach Trail

Harbor Creek

Snow Valley Peak

Secret Harbor

Canyon Road

North Canyon

Secret

Bliss

HUMBOLDT TOIYABE NATIONAL FOREST

Skunk Harbor Trail

Creek

North Canyon

To Carson City

Skunk Harbor

Marlette Lake Trail

Road

Clear Creek

LAKE TAHOE NEVADA STATE PARK

North

Wildcat Cabin

Prey Meadows

Canyon

Canyon

28

Spencers Cabin

Spooner Lake Cabin

Kings

Carson City
Douglas County

Slaughterhouse

Entrance Station

P

Spooner Lake

P

Spooner Summit

50

Spooner Summit

Glenbrook

0   .25   .5   .75   1 mile
0   .5   1 kilometer

To South Lake Tahoe

White Hill

Tahoe Rim Trail

Tahoe Rim Trail: Spooner Summit to Snow Valley Peak

Views of Lake Tahoe from Snow Valley Peak are stunning. However, you'll have to journey through 4 miles of dense forest before the lake is revealed in all its glory. A trio of vista points within the first 2.25 miles offers limited views for those who prefer a shorter hike, but they fail to compare to the awesome grandeur at the trip's climax.

Best Time

Considering the shady forest that this section of the Tahoe Rim Trail (TRT) passes through, one might get the impression that the previous winter's snowpack would hang around well into summer. However, because considerably less snow falls on the Carson Range than the Sierra Crest to the west, this trail opens up sooner than might be expected. In most years hikers can anticipate snow-free hiking beginning in June. The downside is that, by midsummer, very little water, if any, will be available en route to Snow Valley Peak. The cooler clime of autumn makes for pleasant hiking, particularly when the aspens in North Canyon are ablaze with color.

Finding the Trail

Drive on US 50 to Spooner Summit, 0.75 mile east of the junction of NV 28. Parking is available in the well-signed TRT parking lot on the north side of the highway.

TRAIL USE
Hike, Run, Horses, Dogs Allowed

LENGTH
12.4 miles, 7 hours

VERTICAL FEET
±2,900

DIFFICULTY
− 1 2 3 **4** 5 +

TRAIL TYPE
Out-and-back

SURFACE TYPE
Dirt

FEATURES
Mountain
Summit
Autumn Colors
Birds
Cool & Shady
Great Views
Photo Opportunity

FACILITIES
Restrooms
Picnic Tables

Trail Description

▶1 A short mild climb from the parking lot leads into light Jeffrey pine and red fir forest past a junction with a lateral to Spooner Lake. Beyond this junction, the grade of ascent becomes moderate and the forest cover increases. Sporadic gaps in the trees allow brief, partial glimpses of Spooner Lake below, but the majority of the first 4 miles of trail passes through thick forest. At 1.3 miles from the trailhead, a 4- by 4-inch post marks a short lateral leading to a vista point, which offers a view to the east of US 50 winding down Clear Creek Canyon. ▶2

Continue the steady ascent, curving around minor hills and ridges. At 0.6 mile from the previous junction, you reach a second junction, marked by a 4- by 4-inch post, with a lateral to a viewpoint. The short path leads to a boulder-covered knoll and views of Carson Valley to the east and peaks in Desolation Wilderness above Lake Tahoe to the southwest. ▶3

Back on the TRT, proceed on a northbound course through moderate forest cover. After a while the trail veers west and you climb to the crest of a ridge, where, 2.3 miles from the trailhead, another 4- by 4-inch post signals a junction with another lateral to a viewpoint. Follow the lateral for a few hundred feet and then scramble over boulders to a hilltop view of Lake Tahoe. ▶4

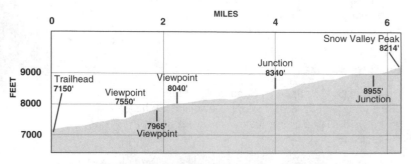

TRAIL 43   TRT: Spooner Summit to Snow Valley Peak
Elevation Profile

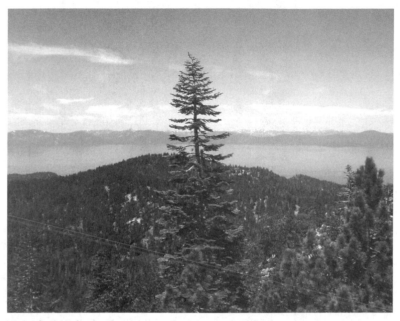

View *of Lake Tahoe*

From the junction, the TRT loosely follows the crest of the Carson Range for the next 1.75 miles, on a more gently graded ascent through mixed forest cover. At 4 miles from the trailhead, you encounter a junction with a 1.2-mile-long trail connecting with the North Canyon Road, which is 700 vertical feet below. ▶5

Proceeding toward Snow Valley Peak, a mild climb leads away from the junction, passing through open terrain on the east side of the ridge, which allows views of Carson Valley and the Pine Nut Mountains. After a switchback, the trail shifts to the west side of the ridge, where Lake Tahoe and the surrounding peaks spring into view, an ample reward for the previous miles of viewless hiking. A few groves of conifers interrupt the views temporarily, but soon you break out into the open for good, following an angling ascent across a hillside carpeted with tobacco brush, sagebrush, and bitterbrush. The views of the Lake Tahoe Basin are quite impressive. Rather than heading directly toward the summit, the TRT climbs steadily toward a saddle directly northwest of it. In this saddle, 5.8 miles from the trailhead, you reach a junction with the old Snow Valley Peak jeep road. ▶6

Turn right, briefly follow the old road, and then turn right again onto an old track heading toward the summit of Snow Valley Peak. After a winding 0.4-mile climb, you reach the 9,214-foot summit. ▶7 Despite the communication towers and accompanying equipment that occupy the summit, the views are stunning, though the broad topography of Snow Valley Peak requires that you move about to get the best views in all directions. Lake Tahoe is the preeminent gem, with Marlette Lake shimmering in the foreground below. Visible peaks are too numerous to list (be sure to pack along a map to help identify them). To the east are Carson City and Eagle Valley, and to the northeast, Washoe Lake, Washoe Valley, and the Truckee Meadows.

Summit

Great Views

🚶	**MILESTONES**	
▶1	0.0	Start at trailhead
▶2	1.3	Lateral to first viewpoint
▶3	1.9	Lateral to second viewpoint
▶4	2.3	Lateral to third viewpoint
▶5	4.0	Continue straight ahead (north) at junction
▶6	5.8	Turn right (east and then southeast) at Snow Valley Peak jeep road
▶7	6.2	Summit of Snow Valley Peak

Spooner Lake

Spooner Lake was created in the 1850s for use as a millpond when a timber company constructed a dam across Spooner Creek. The dam was rebuilt in 1929 for irrigation purposes. Nowadays, within Lake Tahoe Nevada State Park, recreation has replaced logging and irrigation as the principal activity around Spooner Lake, with hikers, naturalists, picnickers, and anglers flocking to the pleasant surroundings. A nearly level, 1.6-mile path encircles the lake, providing an easy hike complete with interpretive displays, park benches, and superb scenery. The trail passes through diverse plant communities, including Jeffrey pine forest, aspen groves, flower-filled meadows, and sagebrush scrub. The area is also home to a wide range of wildlife.

Best Time

The Spooner Lake section of Lake Tahoe Nevada State Park is open all year, with groomed cross-country ski trails replacing the mountain bike and hiking routes in the winter. The Spooner Lake Trail should be snow-free from May, when wildflowers begin their bloom, through October, when stands of aspen turn golden-yellow.

Finding the Trail

Drive on NV 28 to the entrance into the Spooner Lake section of Lake Tahoe Nevada State Park, 1 mile northwest of the junction with US 50. Follow the access road to the visitor center parking lot.

TRAIL USE
Hike, Run, Handicapped Accessible, Dogs Allowed, Child Friendly

LENGTH
1.8 miles, 1 hour

VERTICAL FEET
Negligible

DIFFICULTY
− 1 2 3 4 5 +

TRAIL TYPE
Loop

SURFACE TYPE
Dirt

FEATURES
Mountain
Lake
Autumn Colors
Wildflowers
Birds
Wildlife
Photo Opportunity
Historical Interest

FACILITIES
Restrooms
Picnic Tables
Water
Phone
Visitor Center

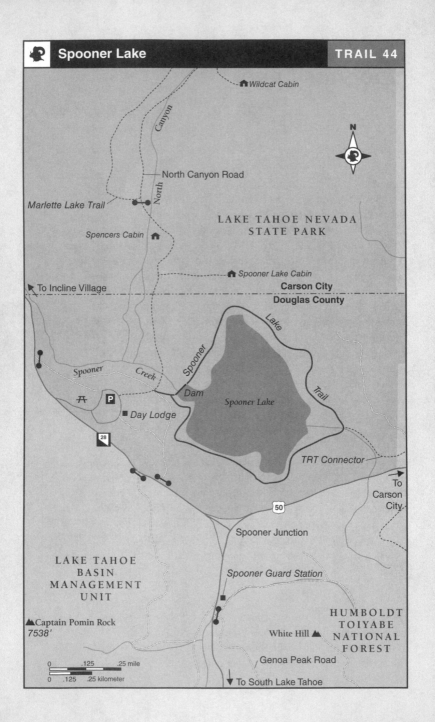

Spooner Lake   TRAIL 44

N

Wildcat Cabin

Canyon

North Canyon Road

North

Marlette Lake Trail

Spencers Cabin

LAKE TAHOE NEVADA
STATE PARK

Spooner Lake Cabin

To Incline Village

Carson City
Douglas County

Lake

Spooner

Creek

Spooner

Dam

Spooner Lake

Trail

Day Lodge

28

TRT Connector

To
Carson
City

50

Spooner Junction

LAKE TAHOE
BASIN
MANAGEMENT
UNIT

Spooner Guard Station

HUMBOLDT
TOIYABE
NATIONAL
FOREST

White Hill

Captain Pomin Rock
7538'

Genoa Peak Road

0   .125   .25 mile

To South Lake Tahoe

0   .125   .25 kilometer

To use an alternate trailhead, drive on US 50 to Spooner Summit, 0.75 mile east from the junction with NV 28, and park on the north side of the road in the Tahoe Rim Trail (TRT) parking lot. Follow the TRT north for approximately 50 yards to an informal junction. Turn left, leaving the TRT, and descend on a lateral, initially paralleling US 50. After 0.75 mile from the TRT Trailhead, you reach a junction with the Spooner Lake Trail on the east side of the lake.

Logistics

Though mountain biking is perhaps the most popular form of recreation within the park, the Spooner Lake Trail is open to pedestrians only. Pets must be leashed. Fishing is catch-and-release only, with mandatory use of barbless artificial lures. A $10 fee is charged for entry into the park.

Trail Description

▶1 A short walk from the parking lot leads to a signed, four-way junction. ▶2 Following directions to Spooner Lake, you stroll past a signboard and begin a clockwise loop around the lake by passing over the dam. Interpretive signs placed around the loop provide opportunities to learn tidbits about the human and natural history of the area. Conveniently placed park benches provide ample opportunities to rest and enjoy the lake views. Circling the lake, you encounter a variety of vegetation: Large clearings are filled with sagebrush, bitterbrush, and mule-ears. Where the soil is able to hold onto more moisture, you'll see pockets of willows. Away from the lakeshore are thick stands of Jeffrey pine forest, interspersed with a smattering of white fir. Near the inlet, dense aspen groves shimmer with a splash of grayish green in summer and a blaze of yellow-gold in fall.

 Historical Interest

 Autumn Colors

On the southeast side of the lake, you reach a junction with the lateral on the left that climbs up to the Tahoe Rim Trailhead near Spooner Summit. ►3 Veer right here and proceed to a wood bridge across Spooner Creek. Beyond the bridge, the trail draws closer to the lakeshore and passes through a flower-filled meadow, which provides a fine habitat **Birds**  for several species of birds, including osprey, bald eagle, and killdeer. Continue around the lake to close the loop at the junction. ►4 From there, follow the short trail back to the parking lot. ►5

🚶	**MILESTONES**	
►1	0.0	Start at trailhead
►2	0.1	Junction with North Canyon Road
►3	1.2	Veer right at junction
►4	1.7	Return to junction with North Canyon Road
►5	1.8	Return to trailhead

Marlette Lake

The trip to Marlette Lake via the North Canyon Road is still a favorite with mountain bikers. (If you're interested in mountain biking, see Trail 46: Flume Trail.) After the 2006 completion of the Marlette Lake Trail, which roughly parallels the road, hikers and equestrians now have their very own route to follow. The 4.5-mile journey starts at one artificial lake, Spooner, and ends at another, Marlette. In between, the trail passes through mixed forest up North Canyon, before a short descent leads to the scenic lakeshore. Once there, hikers, bikers, and equestrians with extra time and energy have additional opportunities to reach fine Lake Tahoe views, colorful wildflower displays, and extensive stands of aspens.

Best Time

The trail to Marlette Lake is generally open for snow-free travel by June. Fall is an especially fine time for a visit, when the extensive aspen groves in North Canyon and along Marlette's west shore are ablaze in autumnal splendor.

Finding the Trail

Drive on NV 28 to the entrance into the Spooner Lake section of Lake Tahoe Nevada State Park, 1 mile northwest of the junction with US 50. Proceed past the fee station ($10 in 2015) to an intersection and veer left into the picnic area parking lot. A right-hand turn leads shortly to a parking lot for the bike rental shop, where a limited selection of food and beverages is available.

TRAIL USE
Hike, Run, Horses,
Dogs Allowed (on leash)
LENGTH
9.0 miles, 4–5 hours
VERTICAL FEET
+1,200/-400
DIFFICULTY
- 1 2 **3** 4 5 +
TRAIL TYPE
Out-and-back
SURFACE TYPE
Dirt

FEATURES
Canyon
Mountain
Stream
Lake
Autumn Colors
Wildflowers
Birds
Wildlife
Photo Opportunity

FACILITIES
Restrooms
Picnic Tables
Concessions

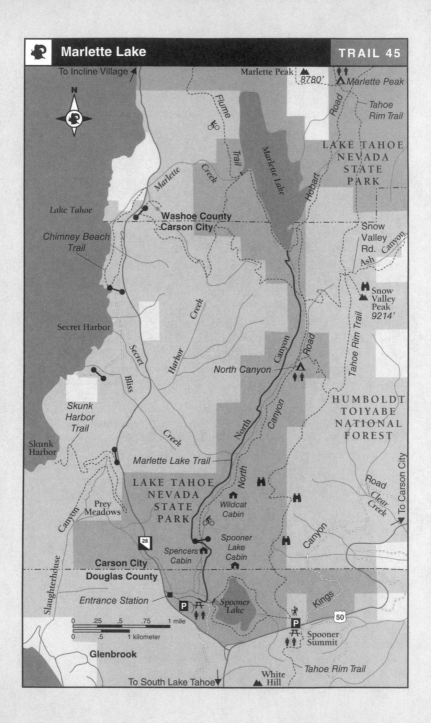

Marlette Lake

TRAIL 45

To Incline Village

Marlette Peak ▲ 8780'

👫 ▲ Marlette Peak

Tahoe Rim Trail

Flume

Trail

Marlette Creek

Marlette Lake

Hobart Road

LAKE TAHOE NEVADA STATE PARK

N

Lake Tahoe

Marlette

Creek

Washoe County Carson City

Chimney Beach Trail

Snow Valley Rd.

Ash Canyon

Secret Harbor

Creek

Secret

Harbor

🅷 Snow Valley Peak 9214' ▲

Bliss

North Canyon

▲ 👫

Canyon

Road

Tahoe Rim Trail

Skunk Harbor Trail

Creek

North

Canyon

HUMBOLDT TOIYABE NATIONAL FOREST

Skunk Harbor

Marlette Lake Trail

🅷

To Carson City →

North

Canyon

Road

Clear Creek

LAKE TAHOE NEVADA STATE PARK

Wildcat Cabin 🏠

Prey Meadows

Canyon

🚲

Spooner Lake Cabin 🏠

🅷

Canyon

Slaughterhouse

28

Spencers Cabin 🏠

Carson City
Douglas County

Entrance Station →

🅿 ⛺ 👫

Spooner Lake

🚶 Kings

🅿 50

⛺ 👫 *Spooner Summit*

0   .25   .5   .75   1 mile
0   .5   1 kilometer

Glenbrook

To South Lake Tahoe ▼

White Hill ▲

Tahoe Rim Trail

Trail Description

►1 From the parking lot, follow signs to all trails through the Jeffrey pine–shaded picnic area and continue on the wide track of a dirt road down a short hill to a four-way junction with a road on the left to a maintenance area and one on the right to Spooner Lake. ►2 Proceed on the gently graded road ahead (northeast) and soon pass around the right-hand edge of an extensive meadow carpeted with grasses and clumps of willow. Shortly beyond the meadow, you reach a junction with a path on the right leading to Spooner Summit Lake Cabin, a hand-hewn Scandinavian-style structure that can sleep up to four adults. The cabin is complete with cooking and heating stoves, kitchen supplies, and an odor-free composting toilet (for rental information, visit **zephyrcove.com/spoonercabins.aspx**). ►3 Remaining on the main road, you pass through a fine grove of aspens and continue to Spencer's Cabin, a structure used by cattlemen in the 1920s. Away from the cabin, the road crosses a piped stream and soon leads to the junction between the continuation of the North Canyon Road and the Marlette Lake Trail. ►4

Veer left and follow singletrack trail through a forest of Jeffrey pines and white firs to a switchback and then continue on a moderate climb up North Canyon, not far to the left of the North Canyon Road. Intermittent breaks in the forest allow limited views to the east of the crest of the Carson Range and, farther up the trail, 9,214-foot Snow Valley Peak. In early summer, these openings in the forest are blessed with a burst of yellow from scads of blooming mule-ears. The moderate ascent is interrupted briefly by a very brief descent to a bridged crossing of a Secret Harbor Creek tributary. About 0.75 mile farther, a series of switchbacks leads farther up the hillside, as you continue a moderate climb up the canyon on the way to a junction with

 Wildflowers

an old road that connects the North Canyon Road (immediately to the right) to the Chimney Beach parking area (3.5 trail miles west). ►5

Remaining on singletrack, you continue ahead from the junction and begin a mild to moderate descent toward the south shore of Marlette Lake, as lodgepole pines and western white pines join the mixed forest. Along the way, the path makes a couple of bridged crossings over the narrow inlet stream before arcing around to a junction with a road near the picturesque lakeshore. ►6 The road follows the southwest shoreline toward the dam and the official start of the Flume Trail. Near the junction is a Nevada Division of Wildlife trout hatchery, built in 1987. Previously closed to anglers, fishing is now allowed for the three resident species—Lahontan cutthroat, rainbow, and brook trout—between July 15 and September 30 (catch and release only). Because the lake is a domestic water source for Carson City, camping is not allowed either, but swimming is permissible, with the water temperature quite refreshing on a typically hot summer day.

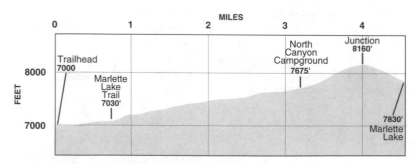

TRAIL 45 Marlette Lake Elevation Profile

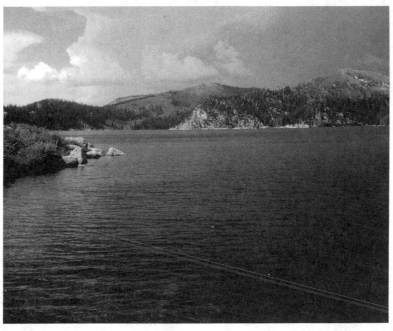

Marlette Lake

🚶 MILESTONES

▶1 0.0 Start at trailhead
▶2 0.1 Continue straight ahead (north) on North Canyon Road
▶3 0.3 Continue straight ahead (north) at Spooner Summit Lake
        Cabin junction
▶4 0.7 Veer left (west) onto Marlette Lake Trail
▶5 4.0 Continue straight ahead (north) at Chimney Beach junction
▶6 4.5 South shore of Marlette Lake

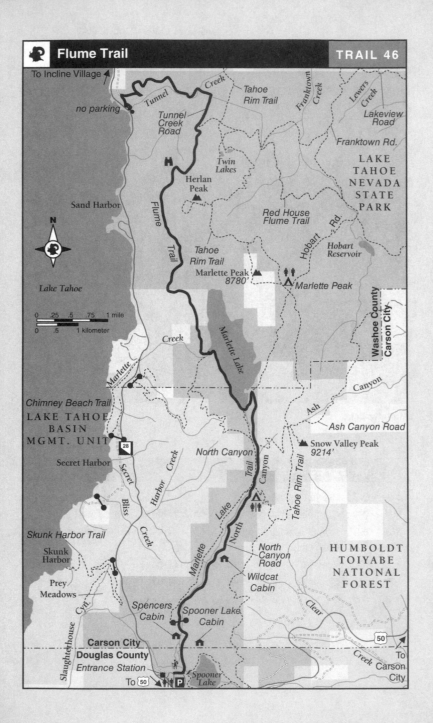

Flume Trail

TRAIL 46

To Incline Village

no parking

Tunnel Creek

Tunnel Creek Road

Tahoe Rim Trail

Franktown Creek

Lewers Creek

Lakeview Road

Franktown Rd.

LAKE TAHOE NEVADA STATE PARK

Sand Harbor

Flume Trail

Twin Lakes

Herlan Peak

Red House Flume Trail

Hobart Rd.

Hobart Reservoir

N

Lake Tahoe

Tahoe Rim Trail

Marlette Peak 8780

Marlette Peak

0   .25   .5   .75   1 mile
0   .5   1 kilometer

Creek

Marlette Lake

Washoe County
Carson City

Marlette Creek

Chimney Beach Trail

LAKE TAHOE BASIN MGMT. UNIT

Ash Canyon

Ash Canyon Road

28

Secret Harbor

Secret Creek

Harbor Creek

North Canyon

Lake North Canyon Trail

Snow Valley Peak 9214'

Tahoe Rim Trail

Bliss Creek

Skunk Harbor Trail

Skunk Harbor

Prey Meadows

Slaughterhouse Cyn.

Marlette Creek

North Canyon Road

North Canyon

Wildcat Cabin

HUMBOLDT TOIYABE NATIONAL FOREST

Spencers Cabin

Spooner Lake Cabin

Clear Creek

50

To Carson City

Carson City
Douglas County
Entrance Station

To 50

Spooner Lake

Flume Trail

The Flume Trail is one of the West's most renowned mountain biking trails, with great views of Lake Tahoe and an easy graded section of singletrack trail combining for Tahoe's ultimate fat-tire excursion. While a stiff climb makes up the first 5 miles, once the incredible views begin the effort is quickly forgotten for the remainder of the downhill romp. All this grandeur does have one drawback—the trail can be quite crowded on sunny summer weekends.

Best Time

The trail is usually snow-free June–October.

Finding the Trail

START: Drive on NV 28 to the entrance into the Spooner Lake section of Lake Tahoe Nevada State Park, 1 mile northwest of the junction with US 50. Proceed past the fee station ($10 in 2015) to an intersection and veer right to the parking lot for the bike rental shop, where, along with bike rentals and repairs, a limited selection of food and beverages is available.

END: Parking is nonexistent anywhere near where the Tunnel Creek Road meets NV 28. Parking along the shoulder of the highway is not allowed in the immediate vicinity, and legal spaces farther along the highway are usually already occupied, especially on a summer weekend. Perhaps the best bet is to bite the bullet and pay for the Flume Trail Shuttle back to Spooner Lake ($15 per person with own bike, free with rental bike). Visit **zephyrcove .com,** or call 775-749-1120 for more information.

TRAIL USE
Bike

LENGTH
13.0 miles, 4 hours

VERTICAL FEET
+1,850/-2,625

DIFFICULTY
– 1 2 **3** 4 5 +

TRAIL TYPE
Point-to-point

SURFACE TYPE
Dirt

FEATURES
Canyon
Mountain
Lake
Autumn Colors
Great Views
Photo Opportunity

FACILITIES
Restrooms
Picnic Tables
Water
Phone
Visitor Center

Logistics

Horses are not permitted on the Flume Trail, and while hikers *are* allowed, the author's recommendation is to leave this trail for mountain bikers.

Not only are mountain bikes available for rent, but reservations can also be made for a pair of backcountry cabins. Both the Spooner Summit Lake Cabin and Wildcat Cabin are hand-hewn Scandinavian-style structures that sleep two to four adults. The cabins are complete with cooking and heating stoves, kitchen supplies, and odor-free composting toilets. Check out the website at **zephyrcove.com /spoonercabins.aspx** to make reservations or for more information.

Trail Description

▶1 From the parking lot follow a wide path for 0.1 mile to a junction with North Canyon Road. ▶2 Head north on a gentle climb across an open area of sagebrush scrub into a mixed forest of lodgepole pines, white firs, and Jeffrey pines, where the grade of ascent increases. Continue a stiff climb through the rolling terrain of North Canyon, amid conifers and aspen groves. At 3.25 miles from the parking lot, a steeper 0.75-mile climb leads to the top of a saddle and the high point of your journey, where

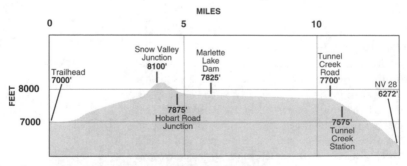

TRAIL 46 Flume Trail Elevation Profile

The Carson Range

The Flume Trail is in the Carson Range, a north–south-trending sub-range of the Sierra Nevada lying to the east of Lake Tahoe. Elevations range from 5,000 feet near the eastern base to 10,881 feet at the summit of Freel Peak. Such a wide elevation spectrum furthers the biological diversity: Dry, sagebrush-covered slopes, common to much of the Great Basin, are present throughout the area, as expected, but so are lush streamside settings more reminiscent of canyons on the west side of the Sierra. Early summer offers hikers a wide array of wildflowers.

The Carson Range holds the most diverse collection of trees in Nevada. In the lower elevations pinyon pines and western junipers intermix with mountain mahoganies. From 5,000 feet to 7,500 feet is the Jeffrey pine–white fir zone, where you'll also find some ponderosa pines, sugar pines, and incense cedars. From 7,500 feet to 9,000 feet is the red fir zone, home to red firs; lodgepole, Jeffrey, and western white pines; white firs; and mountain hemlocks. The upper forest zone, from 9,300 feet to timberline (10,300 feet), features groves of whitebark pines and some lodgepole pines and mountain hemlocks.

The Carson Range is the backyard playground for residents of Reno–Sparks, Carson City, and the Carson Valley towns of Minden and Gardnerville, as well as for visitors and residents of the communities around the east shore of Lake Tahoe. This proximity of urban centers means recreationists will be able to find everything necessary for hiking and backpacking trips into the Carson Range.

roads branch off to Chimney Beach on the left and Snow Valley Peak on the right. ▶3

With the last of the climbing behind, you head downhill toward a well-signed junction with Hobart Road, on the southeast side of scenic Marlette Lake. ▶4 The lake provides an inviting swim if you're still hot from the climb. Turn left and follow the flat road around the south and west sides of the lake. During periods of high water, you may have to carry

 Lake

Lake Tahoe Nevada State Park Bike Trails

Aside from the section of the Tahoe Rim Trail closed to bikes between Spooner Summit and Tunnel Creek Road (Trail 43), options for mountain bikers are many—a fine network of trails and roads carpets the Spooner Backcountry. A full-color brochure, complete with a map showing all the possible routes, is available from Lake Tahoe Nevada State Park, or online at **parks.nv.gov/parks/marlette-hobart-backcountry.**

your bike across some boulders and then across the outlet to reach the start of the Flume Trail proper, near the dam. ▶5

Now on the Flume Trail, you ride pleasantly graded singletrack that makes a mild drop of 40 feet per mile. The trail is narrow and exposed in spots, and you may feel the need to walk your bike across some rockslides, but the stupendous views of Lake Tahoe along the way make the Flume Trail a world-famous ride. The mellow 4.5-mile ride along the Flume Trail ends where the trail merges with Tunnel Creek Road. ▶6

Continue the northbound descent on the road for 0.4 mile to Tunnel Creek Station. ▶7 From there, the steep, sandy road bends west and drops 1,300 feet in 2 miles to NV 28. ▶8

MILESTONES

▶1	0.0	Start at trailhead
▶2	0.1	Head north on North Canyon Road
▶3	4.0	Continue straight ahead (north) at junction for Chimney Beach and Snow Valley Peak
▶4	4.7	Turn left (south) at Hobart Road junction
▶5	6.1	Marlette Lake Dam and start of Flume Trail
▶6	10.5	Merge with Tunnel Creek Road
▶7	10.9	Tunnel Creek Station
▶8	13.0	NV 28

Tahoe Rim Trail: Spooner Summit to South Camp Peak

Lake Tahoe is considered the premier natural wonder in northern Nevada, and this trip to South Camp Peak may provide the quintessential view. Don't forget your camera, as even the most jaded photographer will be impressed by the vistas from the open slopes along the mile-long traverse of the peak. Getting there does require a 5-mile, 1,875-foot climb along a waterless stretch of the Tahoe Rim Trail (TRT), but the scenic rewards are definitely worth the effort.

Best Time

Receiving roughly half the amount of winter snow that falls on Desolation Wilderness, trails in the Carson Range open sooner than their western counterparts. Consequently, in average years, hikers can hit the trail to South Camp Peak by June and continue through October before the first significant snowfall dusts the range.

Finding the Trail

Follow US 50 to Spooner Summit, 0.75 mile east of the junction with NV 28. Park on the south side of the highway in the Spooner Summit picnic area, which has pit toilets.

Logistics

A couple of cautions are worth mentioning. Water is not available along the entire route of the trail—make sure you're carrying a sufficient amount for

TRAIL USE
Hike, Run, Bike,
Horses, Dogs Allowed

LENGTH
10.2 miles, 4–6 hours

VERTICAL FEET
±2,100

DIFFICULTY
– 1 2 **3** 4 5 +

TRAIL TYPE
Out-and-back

SURFACE TYPE
Dirt

FEATURES
Mountain
Summit
Wildflowers
Great Views
Photo Opportunity

FACILITIES
Restrooms

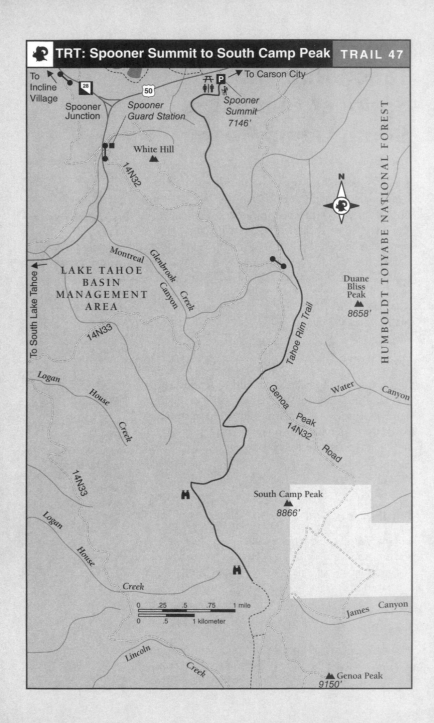

To Incline Village

Spooner Junction

28

50

Spooner Guard Station

To Carson City

P

Spooner Summit 7146'

14N32

White Hill

N

To South Lake Tahoe

Montreal

Glenbrook Creek

Canyon

LAKE TAHOE BASIN MANAGEMENT AREA

14N33

HUMBOLDT TOIYABE NATIONAL FOREST

Duane Bliss Peak 8658'

Logan

House

Creek

Tahoe Rim Trail

Genoa Peak

14N32 Road

Water Canyon

14N33

South Camp Peak 8866'

Logan

House

Creek

0   .25   .5   .75   1 mile
0   .5   1 kilometer

James Canyon

Lincoln

Creek

Genoa Peak 9150'

both the hike in and the hike out. Hikers should maintain a cautious eye while on the trail, as mountain bikes are permitted on this section of the TRT.

Water is not available along the entire route of the trail.

Trail Description

▶1 Leave the trailhead parking lot and make a stiff, switchbacking climb on sandy trail up the hillside south of US 50 through sagebrush, tobacco brush, currant, chinquapin, and manzanita, beneath scattered Jeffrey pines and quaking aspens that dot the slope. Eventually the roar of traffic from the highway is left behind, as you gain a ridge and follow a milder climb along the crest. Farther on, keen eyes will reveal that this area was selectively logged at some time in the past, the result of a bark beetle infestation that killed a number of trees in the early 1990s. This scattered forest of Jeffrey pines and red firs allows partial views of Carson Valley to the east and Lake Tahoe to the west, and provides enough sunlight for a fine array of early summer wildflowers, including mule-ears, lupine, and paintbrush. Near the 1.5-mile mark, you climb to a knoll, where a very short use trail leads to impressive views.

 Wildflowers

 Great Views

A stretch of mild descent, followed by a mild climb, brings you to a crossing of a dirt road,

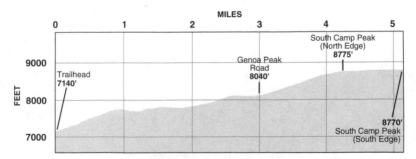

TRAIL 47 TRT: Spooner Summit to South Camp Peak Elevation Profile

2.5 miles from the trailhead. A mildly rising traverse leads across the selectively logged slope below Duane Bliss Peak. At 0.25 mile past the first road crossing, you cross an abandoned road and climb to the crest again. A moderate climb along the ridge takes you just below a rocky knob, where a short use trail leads up the knob to good views of the Carson Valley backdropped by the Pine Nut Range. You eventually leave the views behind, following a mildly graded descent into a mixed forest of western white pines, Jeffrey pines, and red firs to the signed crossing of the Genoa Peak Road (Forest Route 14N32), 3 miles from the trailhead. ►2 This road is a major backcountry thoroughfare for not only the four-wheel-drive crowd but mountain bikers as well.

A moderate climb away from the Genoa Peak Road passes through an area of selective logging and slash burning that is a bit unsightly, though **Wildflowers** ❀ this activity has produced a fine wildflower display in early summer. The long, steady climb reaches a switchback, beyond which the trail bends east before curving back toward the southwest. As you gain elevation, mountain hemlocks and lodgepole pines join the dense, mixed forest. Nearing the crest at the north end of South Camp Peak, approximately 1.3 miles from Genoa Peak Road, you suddenly break out of the forest into a sublime Tahoe vista. ►3 A short climb takes you up to the top of a rocky knoll, where an even better view awaits. Be sure you pack along a detailed map of the Tahoe Basin to help identify the bounty of landmarks visible from this exceptional viewpoint, from where a finer view of the lake is hard to imagine.

The essentially flat-topped plateau of South Camp Peak stretches south for another mile, providing nearly continuous, stupendous lake views. The true summit is actually 0.7 mile east of the trail, hardly worth the extra effort of a cross-country journey. The high point along the trail is another 0.8 mile south, near where a conveniently placed log bench offers an excellent seat for perhaps Tahoe's best show. ▶4

 Summit

![icon]	**MILESTONES**	
▶1	0.0	Start at trailhead
▶2	3.0	Genoa Peak Road
▶3	4.3	North edge of South Camp Peak
▶4	5.1	South edge of South Camp Peak

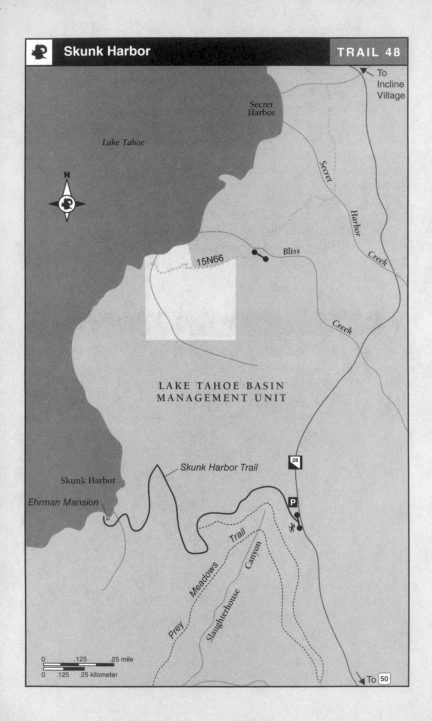

To
Incline
Village

Secret
Harbor

Lake Tahoe

N

15N66

Bliss

Secret

Harbor

Creek

Creek

LAKE TAHOE BASIN
MANAGEMENT UNIT

Skunk Harbor Trail

28

P

Skunk Harbor

Ehrman Mansion

Trail

Meadows

Canyon

Prey

Slaughterhouse

0   .125   .25 mile

0   .125   .25 kilometer

To 50

Skunk Harbor

Lake Tahoe is world renowned for the beauty of its exceptionally clear waters and sparkling sand beaches. Despite its name, Skunk Harbor confirms that reputation, beckoning swimmers, sunbathers, picnickers, and sightseers to visit the scenic, crescent-shaped shoreline. Along with the natural beauty, visitors will experience a bit of history from the Newhall Mansion, a preserved relic from Tahoe's resort period of the early 1900s. The 1.6-mile hike and limited parking at the trailhead ensures that Skunk Harbor won't be as crowded as other Tahoe beaches. Nevertheless, don't expect to be alone.

Best Time

The lake-level elevation ensures a long hiking season, from April to November, but unless you're a card-carrying member of the polar bear club, don't plan to swim in the typically frigid waters of Lake Tahoe unless summer temperatures are prevalent.

Finding the Trail

The trailhead is on the west shoulder of NV 28 at a closed steel gate, 2.4 miles north of the junction with US 50.

TRAIL USE
Hike, Run, Bike, Child Friendly
LENGTH
3.2 miles, 2–3 hours
VERTICAL FEET
±700
DIFFICULTY
– 1 2 **3** 4 5 +
TRAIL TYPE
Out-and-back
SURFACE TYPE
Dirt

FEATURES
Shore
Wildflowers
Great Views
Photo Opportunity
Historical Interest

FACILITIES
Restrooms
Picnic Tables
Water
Phone

OPTION

Side Trip to Prey Meadows

The old railroad grade provides a gently descending route to Prey Meadows, a fine destination in late spring, when copious wildflowers are blooming.

Logistics

Reaching the trailhead may be the most formidable challenge of this trip, as the trailhead is unsigned, parking is extremely limited, and there is no mass transit service available.

Trail Description

▶1 From the highway, descend northwest on a paved road, which quickly turns to dirt, amid Jeffrey pines and white firs, with an understory of manzanita, sagebrush, chinquapin, rabbitbrush, buckwheat, tobacco brush, and wild rose. Lupine and mule-ears brighten the slopes in season. Soon the road curves above the head of Slaughterhouse Canyon and proceeds in a more westerly direction. Keen eyes may spy the old railroad grade hugging the hillside below the road. Built in 1875, the narrow gauge railroad hauled timber to sawmills near Glenbrook. The resulting lumber was primarily used in Virginia City and the mines of the Comstock Lode. A half mile from the highway, the trail intersects the railroad grade. ▶2

Continue on the main road on a steeper, curving descent toward the lake. As you near the shoreline, cedars join the increasingly dense forest, and the

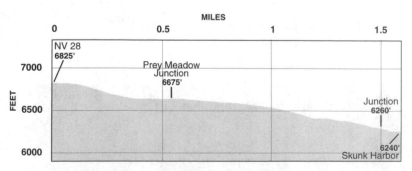

TRAIL 48 Skunk Harbor Elevation Profile

Newhall Mansion

HISTORY

George Newhall built this rustic mansion in 1923 as a wedding present for his wife, Caroline. The property served as a retreat and entertainment center for family and friends until its sale in 1937 to George Whittell. Eventually the property was acquired by the U.S. Forest Service and made accessible for public enjoyment. A number of plaques with photographs provide insights into the history of the area.

underbrush thickens as well. At 1.5 miles, you reach a three-way junction. ▶3 The road to the right leads to the north side of Skunk Harbor's sandy beach, which is bordered by a pile of large rocks. ▶4

Turning left, you cross a tiny stream and parallel the creek toward the lakeshore. Soon the roof and rear walls of the Newhall Mansion appear, along with a patio complete with an outdoor fireplace. Granite steps lead down to the structure, and though the doors are locked, you can peer through iron screens over the windows for a view of the inside. The front porch overlooks the sandy beach and the sparkling clear waters of Skunk Harbor.

Keen eyes may spot the old railroad grade hugging the hillside below the road to Skunk Harbor.

Historical Interest

★	MILESTONES	
▶1	0.0	Start at trailhead
▶2	0.5	Junction with old railroad grade to Prey Meadows
▶3	1.5	Veer left at three-way junction
▶4	1.6	Reach Skunk Harbor

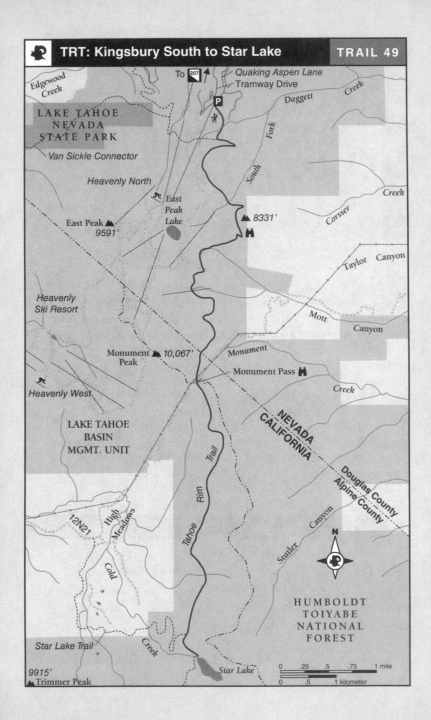

Edgewood Creek

To 207

Quaking Aspen Lane
Tramway Drive

Daggett Creek

P

LAKE TAHOE
NEVADA
STATE PARK

South Fork

Van Sickle Connector

Heavenly North

East Peak Lake

Creek

East Peak 9591'

8331'

Corsser Creek

Taylor Canyon

Heavenly Ski Resort

Mott Canyon

Monument Peak 10,067'

Monument

Monument Pass

Creek

NEVADA
CALIFORNIA

LAKE TAHOE
BASIN
MGMT. UNIT

Tahoe Rim Trail

Douglas County
Alpine County

Heavenly West

12N21

High Meadows

Cold

Studler Canyon

N

Star Lake Trail

HUMBOLDT
TOIYABE
NATIONAL
FOREST

Creek

9915'
Trimmer Peak

Star Lake

0   .25   .5   .75   1 mile

0   .5   1 kilometer

Tahoe Rim Trail: Kingsbury South to Star Lake

Though not the shortest route to lovely Star Lake, this trip offers fine views of Carson Valley and Lake Tahoe away from the crowds. The 17.6-mile round-trip makes for a long day but helps to reduce the number of people you're apt to meet along the way. Once you surmount the first 0.5 mile of steep trail, the remainder is one of the most pleasantly graded sections along the entire 165-mile Tahoe Rim Trail.

Best Time

Hiking season begins in earnest once the winter snows have melted, usually by sometime in June. Mid-July–August will see the warmest temperatures and would be the best time for a dip in lovely Star Lake. Cool but pleasant weather generally lasts from mid-September to the end of October, about when the first significant storm of the season drops snow on the mountains.

Finding the Trail

Drive on NV 207, also known as Kingsbury Grade Road, to Daggett Pass and turn south onto Tramway Drive, which eventually becomes a one-way road that circles through the Nevada side of Heavenly Ski Resort. Park your vehicle in the parking lot near the base of the Stagecoach Express ski lift, 1.5 miles from NV 207. The trailhead has no facilities.

TRAIL USE
Hike, Run, Bike,
Horses, Dogs Allowed

LENGTH
17.6 miles, 10 hours

VERTICAL FEET
±3,500

DIFFICULTY
– 1 2 3 **4** 5 +

TRAIL TYPE
Out-and-back

SURFACE TYPE
Dirt

FEATURES
Mountain
Lake
Great Views
Photo Opportunity
Camping
Secluded

FACILITIES
Restrooms
Picnic Tables

Logistics

Star Lake is an excellent overnight destination, and wilderness permits are not required.

Combining this trip with Trail 50 can create a nice point-to-point trip, though that requires a somewhat lengthy car shuttle.

Trail Description

▶1 Amid towering condominiums and ski area development, the Kingsbury South lateral to the Tahoe Rim Trail (TRT) begins near the base of the Stagecoach Express ski lift and follows a moderate climb up a forested hillside for 0.5 mile, crossing a tributary of South Fork Daggett Creek on the way to a junction with the main trail. ▶2 Turn left (east) at the junction and continue climbing, switchbacking your way to a saddle near a ski area maintenance road, about 1.1 miles from the trailhead and directly southwest of Peak 8,331.

Now through lighter forest, which permits a ground cover of pinemat manzanita, tobacco brush, and chinquapin, you follow mildly graded trail past an informal junction with a short spur to a ski area road and then pass below another chairlift and ski slope. Shortly past the ski slope, hop across the

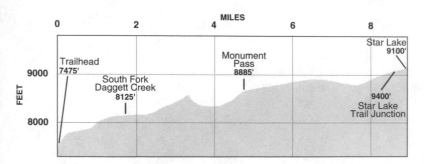

TRAIL 49 TRT: Kingsbury South to Star Lake Elevation Profile

narrow channel of South Fork Daggett Creek, 1.6 miles from the trailhead.

A short, mildly rising traverse leads to a crossing of a jeep road and more views of Carson Valley. Back into the forest, a mile-long, switchbacking climb climaxes at a saddle near Peak 8,611, 3.0 miles from the trailhead, where the trail merges with a ski-area road from East Peak Lake. Just before the saddle you have a fine vista across an open slope of 10,067-foot Monument Peak, 1 mile south-southwest, and the more distant Freel Peak, Jobs Peak, and Jobs Sister.

Descend very steeply along the road toward the bottom of Mott Canyon and curve around to where you'll be grateful as singletrack trail resumes. A short way after the resumption of trail, step over trickling Mott Canyon Creek, which by late summer is usually dry at this elevation, and pass below another Heavenly chairlift. A moderate climb leads out of the canyon, followed by a rising traverse that follows the folds and creases of the topography before angling directly across a mostly open slope. Along the traverse you have expansive eastward views of the Carson Valley, and views to the south of Jobs Peak. Cross the unsigned Nevada–California border and continue the climb to the crest of the Carson Range at Monument Pass, where you meet a junction with the Monument Pass Trail, 3.7 miles from the trailhead. ▶3 Aside from the power lines that run through the pass, the view of Freel Peak and Jobs Sister is quite dramatic, made even better by a short scramble to a neighboring rock outcrop.

Now on the west side of the crest, follow sandy trail on an open, 2-mile traverse through widely scattered trees with good views down into High Meadows and across the lake to the Crystal Range peaks in Desolation Wilderness. On a nearly imperceptible descent, you eventually enter a light forest that obscures most of the views. At 7.7 miles, you encounter the flower-lined, refreshing brook of a

Though not the shortest route to lovely Star Lake, this trip offers fine views of Carson Valley and Lake Tahoe away from the crowds.

 Great Views

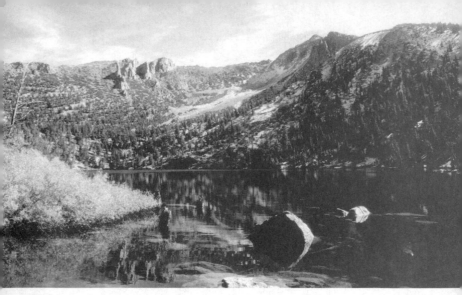

Star Lake *and Jobs Sister (right)*

Lake 〰

Cold Creek tributary. From there, the slightly rising trail proceeds through western white pines, mountain hemlocks, and lodgepole pines toward Star Lake. At 8.6 miles you reach a junction with the Star Lake Trail heading west. ►4 Just before the lake, the trail curves east and then drops to a crossing of the outlet. ►5

At 9,100 feet, Star Lake is one of the highest lakes in the Tahoe Basin, and therefore not one of the warmest. A number of passable campsites along the north shore lure overnighters.

🚶	MILESTONES	
►1	0.0	Start at trailhead
►2	0.5	Turn left at TRT junction
►3	3.7	Monument Pass/junction with Cold Creek Trail
►4	8.6	Star Lake Trail junction
►5	8.8	Star Lake

Tahoe Rim Trail: Armstrong Pass to Star Lake

This trip leads to two excellent destinations, Freel Peak, the highest summit in the Tahoe Basin, and Star Lake, one of the basin's highest lakes. A lightly used section of the Tahoe Rim Trail (TRT) takes you all the way to the lake, and most of the way to the summit. The remainder of the climb to Freel Peak follows a recently improved trail to the top, suitable for all but the most timid of trail hikers. Backdropped by the volcanic slopes of rugged Jobs Sister, the lake's setting is quite picturesque, luring both day hikers and backpackers to the serene shores. The view from Freel Peak is stunning in both scenery and scope.

Best Time

The route along the TRT to Star Lake is often open by the Fourth of July, but those wishing to climb Freel Peak will most likely find snowfields still covering the slopes below the summit at that time. Snow-free ascents of the peak are usually possible by the end of July. The high elevation of Star Lake ensures chilly swimming throughout the season, but the warmer temperatures mid-July–August make a dip in the lake more palatable. Though cooler temperatures prevail in autumn, you'll find less traffic on the trail. Snow returns to the area by late October.

Finding the Trail

From CA 89, turn north onto Forest Route 051, 0.8 mile from the CA 88 junction in Hope Valley and 1.8 miles from Luther Pass. Follow the

TRAIL USE
Hike, Run, Bike,
Horses, Dogs Allowed

LENGTH
12.8 miles, 6–7 hours

VERTICAL FEET
±2,200

DIFFICULTY
– 1 2 **3** 4 5 +

TRAIL TYPE
Out-and-back

SURFACE TYPE
Dirt

FEATURES
Mountain
Summit
Lake
Great Views
Photo Opportunity
Camping

FACILITIES
None

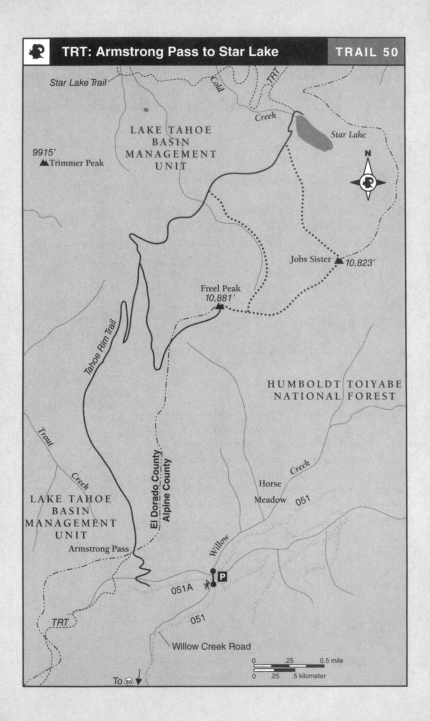

Star Lake Trail

Cold

TRT

Creek

LAKE TAHOE
BASIN
MANAGEMENT
UNIT

Star Lake

N

9915'
▲Trimmer Peak

Jobs Sister ▲ 10,823'

Freel Peak
10,881'
▲

Tahoe Rim Trail

HUMBOLDT TOIYABE
NATIONAL FOREST

Trout

Creek

Creek

LAKE TAHOE
BASIN
MANAGEMENT
UNIT

El Dorado County
Alpine County

Horse

Meadow   051

Armstrong Pass

Willow

051A 🚶 P

051

TRT

Willow Creek Road

0   .25   0.5 mile
0   .25   .5 kilometer

To 89 ▼

sometimes-rough dirt road northwest for nearly 3.5 miles to an intersection with FR 051F on your left, which is blocked to traffic by large boulders (this intersection is immediately after the second bridge over Willow Creek). Park your vehicle nearby as space allows.

Logistics

The dirt road to the trailhead is rough enough to advise the use of a sturdy vehicle with good clearance.

Trail Description

▶1 From the trailhead, proceed on dirt road for a short distance to a flat area just before the rough road makes a steep climb up a low hill. Follow the road for a half-mile to a wide turnaround, where a Tahoe Rim Trail (TRT) sign and an arrow mark the beginning of singletrack trail. Climb moderately steeply, soon crossing a small tributary of Willow Creek. Beyond the crossing, switchbacks attack a hillside carpeted with sagebrush, currant, and tobacco brush and dotted with an occasional western white pine or juniper. At 1.0 mile from the trailhead, the stiff climb ends at a four-way junction at Armstrong Pass, amid scattered red firs. ▶2

Turn right and follow the pleasantly graded TRT on a rising traverse below the west slope of the Carson Range crest. You quickly emerge from the scattered forest and walk across mostly open slopes past an occasional western white pine or juniper. Past a rock cliff known as Fountain Face you enjoy good views across the Trout Creek drainage of the meadows in Hell Hole and Fountain Place, and across Lake Tahoe of the Crystal Range. Continue the steadily rising traverse, hopping over a few tiny rivulets along the way. Near the 3.4-mile mark, the trail angles across the slope via the first of a pair of

 Great Views

Side Trip to Freel Peak

If you're bound for the summit of Freel Peak, leave the Tahoe
Rim Trail (TRT) at the high point of the ridge, 4.6 miles from
the trailhead, ▶3 and head past a sign reading FREEL PEAK 1
on the sandy tread of a trail. In the mid-2000s, the placement
of numerous rock steps and the construction of several short
switchbacks replaced the multiple paths of an old use trail.
The old use trail suffered from erosion and potential damage
to the unique alpine environment of such plants as the unique
Tahoe draba, a low-growing, matted plant with yellow flowers
found only on north- or east-facing slopes in the Freel Peak
and Mount Rose areas. Follow switchbacks up the right-hand
side of a ridge past low rock outcrops before gaining the ridge
crest, with occasional views straight down some precipitous
cliffs. Continue climbing up the ridge until the trail veers left
on an angling ascent across the gravelly northwest face of the
peak to the summit.

In former days an array of communication equipment littered the summit, producing an annoying electronic hum that
would irritate the ears of successful mountaineers. Thankfully,
just about all traces of the man-made equipment have been
removed from the summit area, and nowadays the splendid
vista from the top is no longer tainted by this unsightly and
noisy hindrance. From the top of the Tahoe Basin's highest
summit, the 360-degree unobstructed views of the lake and
the surrounding terrain are truly magnificent.

Peak baggers can easily add 10,823-foot Jobs Sister to
their list of accomplishments by following the mile-long path
along the ridge between Freel Peak and the Tahoe Basin's
second highest summit. More ambitious climbers can triple
summit by heading generally east on a 1.75-mile cross-
country route to 10,633-foot Jobs Peak. Experienced off-trail
hikers bound for Star Lake need not retrace their steps to the
TRT, but rather can descend a use trail down a gully between
Freel Peak and Jobs Sister to the TRT west of the lake, or the
steeper north ridge of Jobs Sister directly to the lakeshore. ▶4
This side trip to Freel Peak adds about 2 miles round-trip and
1,150 vertical feet to the described trail.

long-legged switchbacks. At 4.6 miles, amid scattered whitebark pines, the climb culminates at the crest of an auxiliary ridge of Freel Peak, at 9,730 feet the high point of the trail to Star Lake (and the start of the side trip to Freel Peak). ►3

Remaining on the TRT, descend from the ridge via some switchbacks to the floor of a cirque basin on the northwest side of Freel Peak. A short, moderate descent leads through open forest to the crossing of a thin ribbon of water from a tributary of Cold Creek. Beyond the stream, you follow a nearly mile-long traverse to the north ridge of Jobs Sister, and then make a short drop along the ridge to Star Lake. ►4

At 9,100 feet, Star Lake is one of the highest lakes in the Tahoe Basin, and therefore not one of the warmest. Backpackers will find a number of passable campsites along the north shore with a nice view across the lake of Jobs Sister.

Before construction of the Tahoe Rim Trail, Star Lake was virtually inaccessible. Nowadays, not having a trail to this delightful cirque-bound lake is hard to imagine.

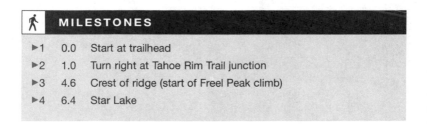

🚶	**MILESTONES**		
►1	0.0	Start at trailhead
►2	1.0	Turn right at Tahoe Rim Trail junction
►3	4.6	Crest of ridge (start of Freel Peak climb)
►4	6.4	Star Lake

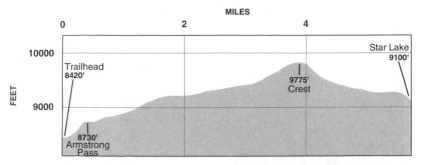

TRAIL 50 TRT: Armstrong Pass to Star Lake Elevation Profile

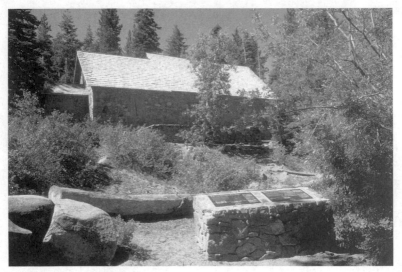

Newhall Mansion (*Trail 48*)

Appendix 1

Top-Rated Trails

North Tahoe

4. Castle Peak
7. Mount Judah Loop
8. Pacific Crest Trail: Donner Pass to Squaw Valley
15. Tahoe Rim Trail: Tahoe Meadows to Brockway Summit

West Tahoe

17. Tahoe Rim Trail: Ward Creek to Twin Peaks
22. Ed Z'berg Sugar Pine Point State Park Nature Trails

South Tahoe

25. Rubicon Trail
26. Vikingsholm and Eagle Falls
31. Mount Tallac
32. Glen Alpine to Susie and Heather Lakes and Lake Aloha
35. Echo Lakes to Lake of the Woods and Ropi Lake

East Tahoe

45. Marlette Lake
46. Flume Trail
47. Tahoe Rim Trail: Spooner Summit to South Camp Peak
48. Skunk Harbor
50. Tahoe Rim Trail: Armstrong Pass to Star Lake

Appendix 2

Local Resources

Major Outfitters

Alpenglow Sports
415 N Lake Tahoe Blvd.
Tahoe City, CA 96145
530-583-6917; **alpenglowsports.com**

The BackCountry
11400 Donner Pass Road
Truckee, CA 96161
530-582-0909; **thebackcountry.net**

Recreational Equipment, Inc. (REI)
2225 Harvard Way
Reno, NV 89502
775-828-9090; **rei.com**

Tahoe Sports Limited
4000 Lake Tahoe Blvd.
South Lake Tahoe, CA 96150
530-542-4000; **tahoesportsltd.com**

Outlets

Patagonia
8550 White Fir St.
Reno, NV 89523
775-746-6878; **patagonia.com**

Sierra Trading Post
6139 B S. Virginia St.
Reno, NV 89502
775-828-8050; **sierratradingpost.com**

Sportif
1415 Greg St., Ste. 101
Sparks, NV 89431
775-353-3434 or 888-357-3567;
sportifoutlet.com

Major Organizations

League to Save Lake Tahoe
530-541-5388; **keeptahoeblue.org**

Tahoe Area Sierra Club
530-320-1795;
motherlode.sierraclub.org/tahoe

Tahoe Rim Trail Association
775-298-4485; **tahoerimtrail.org**

Major Public Agencies

Department of Parks and Recreation
California State Parks
800-777-0369 or 916-653-6995;
www.parks.ca.gov

Eldorado National Forest
530-622-5061;
www.fs.usda.gov/eldorado

Humboldt–Toiyabe National Forest
775-331-6444; **www.fs.usda.gov/htnf**

Carson Ranger District
775-882-2766

Lake Tahoe Basin Management Unit
530-543-2600;
www.fs.usda.gov/ltbmu

Lake Tahoe Nevada State Park
775-831-0494; **parks.nv.gov**

Tahoe National Forest
530-265-4531;
www.fs.usda.gov/tahoe

Big Bend Visitor Center
49685 Hampshire Rocks Rd.
Soda Springs, CA 95728
530-426-3609

Truckee Ranger District
530-587-3558

Appendix 3

Useful Books

Carville, Julie Stauffer. *Hiking Tahoe's Wildflower Trails*. Edmonton, Alberta, Canada: Lone Pine Publishing, 1998.

Graf, Michael. *Plants of the Tahoe Basin: Flowering Plants, Trees, and Ferns*. Los Angeles, CA: University of California Press, 1999.

Hauserman, Tim. *Tahoe Rim Trail: The Official Guide for Hikers, Mountain Bikers, and Equestrians*. 3rd ed. Birmingham, AL: Wilderness Press, 2012.

Lekisch, Barbara. *Tahoe Place Names: The Origin and History of Names in the Lake Tahoe Basin*. Lafayette, CA: Great West Books, 1996.

Schaffer, Jeffrey P. *Desolation Wilderness and the South Lake Tahoe Basin: A Guide to Lake Tahoe's Finest Hiking Area*. 4th ed. Berkeley, CA: Wilderness Press, 2003.

White, Mike. *Afoot and Afield: Reno–Tahoe: A Comprehensive Hiking Guide*. Berkeley, CA: Wilderness Press, 2006.

Appendix 4

Maps

The introduction to each chapter describes U.S. Forest Service and state park maps for that area. Listed below, by chapter, are the names of U.S. Geological Survey (USGS) 7.5-minute quadrangles, plus which trails in this book are shown on that map.

Chapter 1: North Tahoe

Trail 1	Independence Lake, Webber Peak
Trail 2	Hobart Mills
Trail 3	Independence Lake, Norden
Trails 4–5	Norden
Trail 6	Cisco Grove, Soda Springs
Trail 7	Norden
Trails 8–10	Granite Chief, Tahoe City
Trail 11	Tahoe City
Trails 12–14	Mount Rose
Trail 15	Mount Rose, Martis Peak
Trail 16	Mount Rose, Marlette Lake

Chapter 2: West Tahoe

Trail 17	Tahoe City, Homewood
Trails 18–19	Homewood
Trail 20	Bear Pen, Wentworth Springs
Trail 21	Homewood
Trail 22	Meeks Bay

Chapter 3: South Tahoe

Chapter 4: East Tahoe

Index

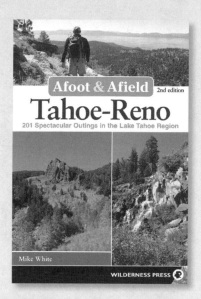

About the Author

Mike White

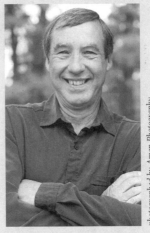

photographed by Amen Photography

Mike White was raised in the suburbs of Portland, Oregon, in the shadow of Mount Hood (whenever the Pacific Northwest skies cleared enough to allow such things as shadows). As a teenager, Mike began hiking, backpacking, and climbing in the Cascades of Oregon and Washington and then honed his outdoor skills while attending Seattle Pacific University.

After acquiring a BA in political science, Mike relocated to Reno, Nevada, with his wife, Robin. In the early 1990s, Mike left his last "real" job (with an engineering firm) and began writing full-time. His first project for Wilderness Press was an update and expansion of Luther Linkhart's classic guide *The Trinity Alps*. His first solo project was *Nevada Wilderness Areas and Great Basin National Park*. He is the author of the popular Snowshoe series; guides to Lassen Volcanic, Kings Canyon, and Sequoia National Parks; as well as guides to the Reno–Tahoe area. Mike has contributed to *Backpacking California, Sierra North*, and *Sierra South* and has written for *Sunset* and *Backpacker* magazines, as well as the *Reno Gazette–Journal*.

Mike taught hiking, backpacking, and snowshoeing classes at a local community college and dispensed trail information while working part-time at REI. He lives in Reno with Robin and their youngest son, Stephen, along with their two labs. David, Mike and Robin's oldest son, still resides in the area.

Joe Walowski

Joe Walowski conceived of the Top Trails series in 2003 and was series editor of the first three titles: *Top Trails Los Angeles, Top Trails San Francisco Bay Area*, and *Top Trails Lake Tahoe*. He currently lives in Seattle.